Mental Health Promotion

What are the first signs of mental distress?

...g mental distress as an illness limits the range of solutions to ...y medical treatments. Most people now recognize that to ...ge it effectively requires a range of approaches that identify and meet the individual needs of the person in distress. For further information about different mental health problems, see Mind's 'Understanding' series of booklets.

The first signs of mental distress will be different for the person in distress and the people around them. When a person's mood starts to change, it may take some time for them to become aware of it. People around them may be more conscious of changes than they are themselves. Changes in sleep patterns are a common sign, and appetite can also be affected. More time spent in bed, allied with lethargy and lower than normal levels of energy, and a reduced desire to socialize are often forerunners of bouts of depression. A reduced need to sleep, an increased desire to go out, and higher levels of energy and creativity are the corresponding indicators of mood highs.

The effects of seeing and/or hearing things others don't, particularly for the first time, can be quite dramatic. Hearing voices can be a very confusing experience. It is often, but not always, apparent that no one else can hear the voices. Sometimes it can be very frustrating that other people cannot hear the voices as well. People are so used to believing what they see that when they see things that others don't, the experience can cause immense distress. It is almost impossible not to react to things that you hear and/or see and this is one of the most frightening aspects of mental distress.

The behaviour of people who are hearing and/or seeing things can be unnerving to those around them. Someone may appear to be talking, or even shouting and swearing, conversing with voices others cannot hear. Some people react to voices by confronting them, this requires a high level of understanding by people closest to them. When someone sees things, their reactions depend on what they are seeing. Some images are so frightening that people just freeze or scream at them. Others may try to hide from what they see. The instinct to escape can be very strong for some, and this can lead to people running away, sometimes flattening anything that gets in their way.

3

How to ... *recognize the early signs of mental distress*

Some people will start to perceive changes in their own body, and others may feel that their body is being controlled by an external force. Some people will react to this feeling by attacking their own body. What may seem to an observer like a suicide attempt, or self injury may be the only way a person can think of ridding themselves of the external control.

Strange or disturbing though these reactions may seem, they do make much more sense if people have some understanding of what the perceptions of the person in distress are. Different outward indications are examined in more detail below.

Am I going mad?

When people first experience mental distress it is not unusual for someone to think that they are going mad. All the stereotypes of insanity, from 'Jekyll and Hyde' to 'Psycho', come flooding to mind and people often start to doubt themselves. They may doubt their ability to think and reason, they may think that they are becoming a danger to those around them, they may have fears about being locked up in an asylum.

These fears – fears that are reinforced by the way the media caricatures 'mental illness' – often prevent someone from talking about things. The risk of being branded mad, of losing friends, and of losing freedom, acts to deter people from being open about their experiences. This in turn increases their own distress and sense of isolation, and adds to the frustration of those around them.

In fact, people's worst fears are unlikely to come true. There are many problems that follow the onset of mental distress, but putting up shutters tends to make things worse. Talking about the experiences and discussing them with people that are trusted tends to be the best way of minimizing the distress. Real friends will be supportive, but they may be unsure about how to respond. They will, over time, learn how best to help. They will also be well-placed to help break down some of the stigma and prejudice that surrounds mental distress.

How can I find out what someone is feeling

When someone starts behaving in a manner that suggests that they may be suffering from mental distress, be sensitive. They may have some or all of the fears outlined above, and need you to do what you can to allay them. Don't be too quick to judge. It is important that a person in distress has someone that they can trust and talk to openly.

Sometimes opening up to relatives is simply impossible. If this is the case, trying to force someone to express their distress is likely to make things worse. People who have had similar experiences are often the easiest to communicate with. There are many local groups – a number run by Mind – that cover the range of different types of mental distress. There are some that offer support for relatives, some for people in distress only, groups for women (or occasionally men) only, groups for people from particular ethnic backgrounds, and some that cover very specific areas. The latter include a number of the relatively new local 'hearing voices' groups.

Finding out about, and offering information on, local groups is a good way of being supportive. The good groups will not impose undue pressure on people, but will offer a degree of understanding that only comes from shared experience. Similarly, relatives/carers groups like those run by the National Schizophrenia Fellowship can offer support and information to people who also feel a sense of frustration and isolation when mental distress strikes. For further information see Helpful organizations.

What causes mental distress

Just as the term mental distress covers a wide range of different experiences, likewise there is an equal range of possible causes. There is some evidence that those forms of distress associated with mood can be linked with changes in brain chemistry. It is not known, however, whether the chemistry causes the mood changes or vice versa. There are many good reasons why people get depressed or elated. It is not very useful to pursue elaborate bio-chemical explanations when there are simple answers to be found in the conditions of a person's life.

How to ... recognize the early signs of mental distress

There are many life events that can contribute to the onset of mental distress. Bereavement is a common trigger – the loss of a loved one is hard on anybody. For many people the effects of grief can be devastating. Whilst hearing or seeing someone who has recently died is not unusual, and a degree of depression is almost inevitable, for some people it can go far beyond bearable limits. The break-up of a relationship can be as damaging as a bereavement. The fall in self-esteem that goes with the end of a relationship can compound that which accompanies mental distress. Criticism from others reinforces self-criticism, which in turn can feed criticism from voices.

For a significant number of people who experience mental distress, problems can be linked back to physical or sexual abuse, sometimes many years prior to the distress. There are other traumas in someone's life that can lead directly, or indirectly to future distress. It should not be surprising that accidents or disasters, or even wars, take their toll in distress for the victims or their loved ones.

There are some forms of distress that can be clearly connected with particular events or incidents. Depression following the birth of a child is widely recognized. Problems with perception can be a result of certain drugs a person has taken years before.

No one really knows why some people hear or see things that others don't, or why some people react to life events far more than others. Explanations range from the hi-tech medical, through the psychological and social, to the religious and spiritual ones. Why someone is hearing or seeing things is almost always less important than how best to cope with the experience. People find, however, that certain events or circumstances can act as triggers for them. Recognizing these triggers, as with identifying sources of extremes of mood, can help minimize both the likelihood of mental distress, and its detrimental effect when it strikes.

Mental Health Promotion

What happens when someone hears 'voices' or sees 'visions'?

The experience of hearing voices is remarkably widespread. Many people hear voices throughout their lives without it causing them any difficulties or distress at all. Some people would be lost without their voices. Different societies treat (or have treated) people who see or hear things in different ways. Generally, however, seeing or hearing things only comes to the attention of others when it becomes a problem.

To understand why someone is behaving as they are, you have to imagine what they are going through, and how you might react in similar circumstances. If, for instance, someone is talking to you, you are likely to answer back. If they are bothering you, you might well ask them, in the strongest terms, to go away. So it is with voices. What appears to be a person ranting, hurling random abuse, or holding a strange one-sided conversation, becomes a reasonable response if you appreciate that they are responding to voices.

The same is true of people who see things. If something frightens you, you might react by freezing. If something appears to be hunting you, you may try to hide, or even run away. If something attacks you, you might try to defend yourself. If it tries to strike you, you may flinch or duck. If something is scary enough, you might just scream. All these reactions are perfectly rational to someone if they perceive something threatening. Only by appreciating what someone is experiencing can you hope to understand the behaviour that goes with it. See Further reading.

Why do people self-harm?

One extreme reaction to different perceptions is self-harm. This is one of the most misunderstood of all aspects of mental distress. Self-harm is often mistaken for either attention-seeking behaviour ('a cry for help'), or as an attempt at suicide. People self-harm for a number of different reasons. Some people see and feel something, a serpent for example, attacking them. You cannot simply run away from something wrapped around your arm. Some people may believe the only way to be free of such an attack is to take a knife to it. For some people self-harm may be a way of controlling feelings of powerlessness and helplessness. Feelings of possession or bodily change can also prompt people to self-harm. Until someone appreciates why an individual is, for example cutting themselves, it is almost impossible to provide constructive support. Dealing with any wounds is obviously a high priority. Dealing with different perceptions takes longer. See Further reading.

How to ... recognize the early signs of mental distress

What other problems might mental distress cause?

Sometimes it is difficult to separate the direct effects of mental distress from the consequences. Depression, for example may be mental distress, or a rational response to hearing critical voices, or seeing frightening things. Loss of sleep may be part of a high mood, or it may be because sleep is impossible for other reasons. A change in appetite or eating habits may be apparent as well.

Many of the problems that accompany mental distress have a knock-on effect on a person's physical health. This can make coping with distress much more difficult. It is important that physical health needs are adequately addressed. If the distressed person remains in good shape physically, the depth and duration of mental distress will almost certainly be reduced.

There is a strong association in the minds of many between mental illness and being dangerous to others. The excessive, and often inaccurate, reporting of acts of violence committed by people with psychiatric diagnoses, particularly schizophrenia, has reinforced this myth. The facts are more reassuring. There are relatively few serious acts of violence committed by people as a result of mental distress. There are, however, things that anyone can do to reduce the risk of danger when someone is in a state of distress. The most important thing is to try and understand why someone may be behaving as they are. If they appear to be trying to escape from something, blocking an escape route is likely to increase risk. If someone is hiding, dragging them out from their refuge may well add to the danger. Above all, calm reactions are more effective than panicked ones.

What can be done when someone starts to experience mental distress?

Some people benefit from talking to other people, others need time to themselves. Trust and respect are important; they help to build and maintain the self-esteem that mental distress can so easily crush. Self-help groups of the type indicated above offer a forum for exchanging coping techniques. There are a number of professionals that may be able to offer a variety of types of support: from informal advice from a family doctor, through counselling and psychotherapy, to drugs from a psychiatrist.

There is no single guaranteed approach, whether spiritual, social or medical. If people are given a range of support, they will be better placed to identify for themselves the types of treatments, therapies, or lifestyles that minimize their own distress.

Mental Health Promotion

There is a strong temptation, possibly more so amongst relatives or carers, to accept an easy explanation, or diagnosis for a state of mental distress. It is often felt that if something is given a medical name then you are halfway to solving the problem. Sadly, this is not the case. Medication can play an important role for some people, while for others it may be no help at all.

Relapse or withdrawal?

For people who have a history of mental distress, there are added complications associated with changes in medication. If someone decides to reduce the amount of medication they are taking, or if they decide to stop altogether, this is likely to have a significant effect on their state of mind. Most drugs prescribed by psychiatrists have potential withdrawal effects. These are sometimes mistaken for signs of a relapse of symptoms.

If someone decides to come off prescribed medication, it is important that they make people around them aware of this. Many people have successfully reduced their medication, or come off it altogether. The best way to succeed is to do it slowly, with as much support as possible from those around you. Changes in mood and perception are common withdrawal effects. They are less likely if withdrawal is slow and paced (up to twelve months or longer would not be unusual), and they are much easier to cope with in a supportive environment. For more detailed information about drugs and advice about withdrawal, see Mind's 'Making Sense of Treatments and Drugs' series of booklets.

Can the effects of mental distress be overstated?

It is part of human nature to try to analyse and explain everything. There is a risk that perfectly normal behaviour will be viewed as an indicator of mental distress, simply because someone has suffered from distress before. People should not look for mental distress, if you examine anyone's conduct closely enough you could find signs of it. The more thoughtful and measured your response, the more effective any interventions are likely to be.

How to ... find out more

Helpful organizations

British Association for Counselling
1 Regent Place, Rugby, Warwickshire CV21 2PJ (01788-578328). Information and advice about counselling and psychotherapy.

Depression Alliance
PO Box 1022, London SE1 7QB (0171-721 7672).

The Hearing Voices Network
Floor 1, Fourways House, 16 Tariff Street, Manchester M1 2EP (0161-228 3896).

Manic Depression Fellowship
8-10 High Street, Kingston-upon-Thames, Surrey KT1 1EY (0181-974 6550).

Mind*info*Line
0181-522 1728 London, 0345-660 163 outside London, Mon-Fri 9.15-4.45.
Wide range of mental health information including access to legal advice.

National Schizophrenia Fellowship
28 Castle Street, Kingston-upon-Thames, Surrey KT1 1SS (0181-547 3937).

Samaritans
0345-90 90 90, 24-hour service.

The Fourth of July

by Natalie Goldstein

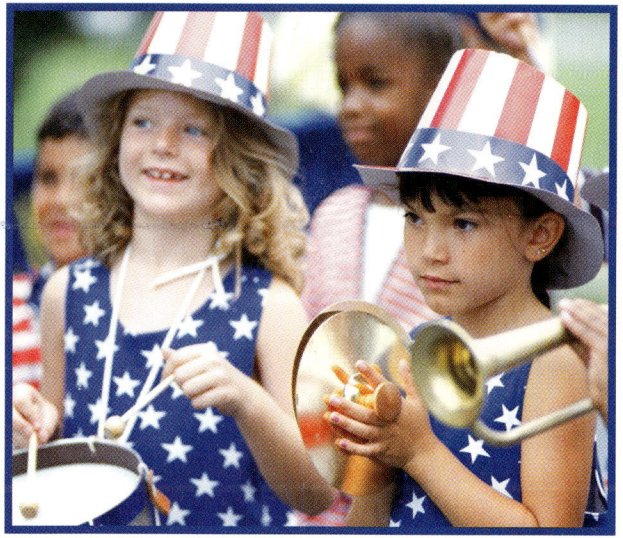

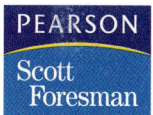

Editorial Offices: Glenview, Illinois • Parsippany, New Jersey • New York, New York
Sales Offices: Needham, Massachusetts • Duluth, Georgia • Glenview, Illinois
Coppell, Texas • Sacramento, California • Mesa, Arizona

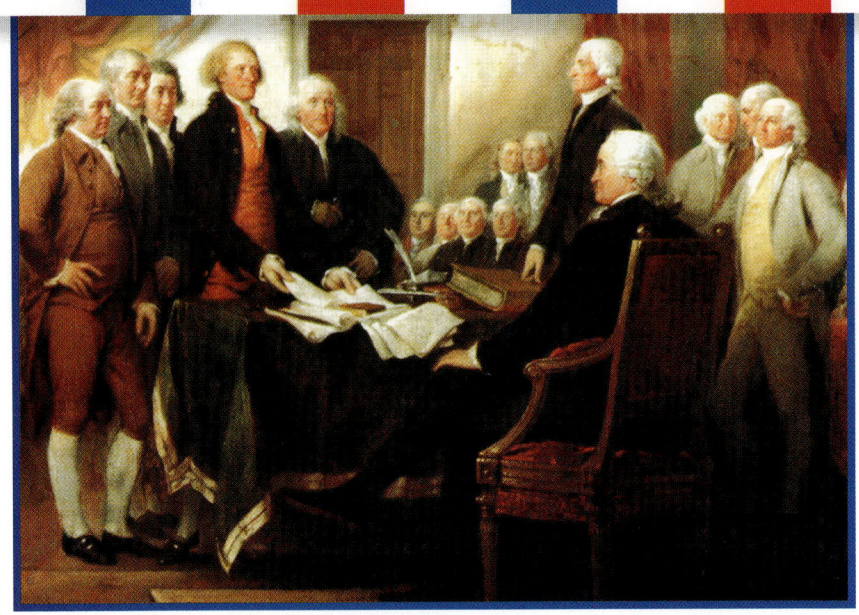

The signing of the Declaration of Independence

The Colonies

Long ago people lived in colonies. The colonies were ruled by England. The colonists wanted **freedom**.

On July 4, 1776, a group of leaders in the colonies agreed on an important paper. It was called the Declaration of Independence.

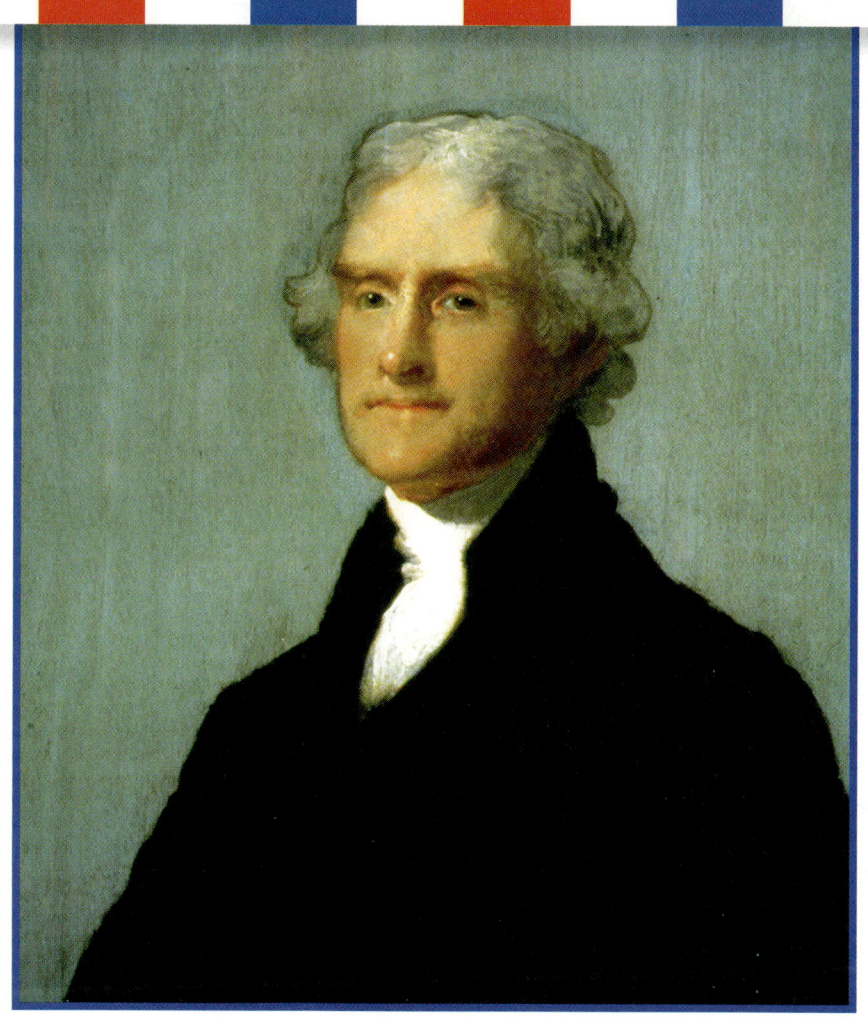

Thomas Jefferson

Most of the Declaration of Independence was written by Thomas Jefferson. July 4 became an American **holiday** to celebrate freedom.

The Fight for Freedom

The colonists had an army to help fight for freedom. George Washington led the army.

The Americans won the war! George Washington became the first **President** of the United States.

George Washington

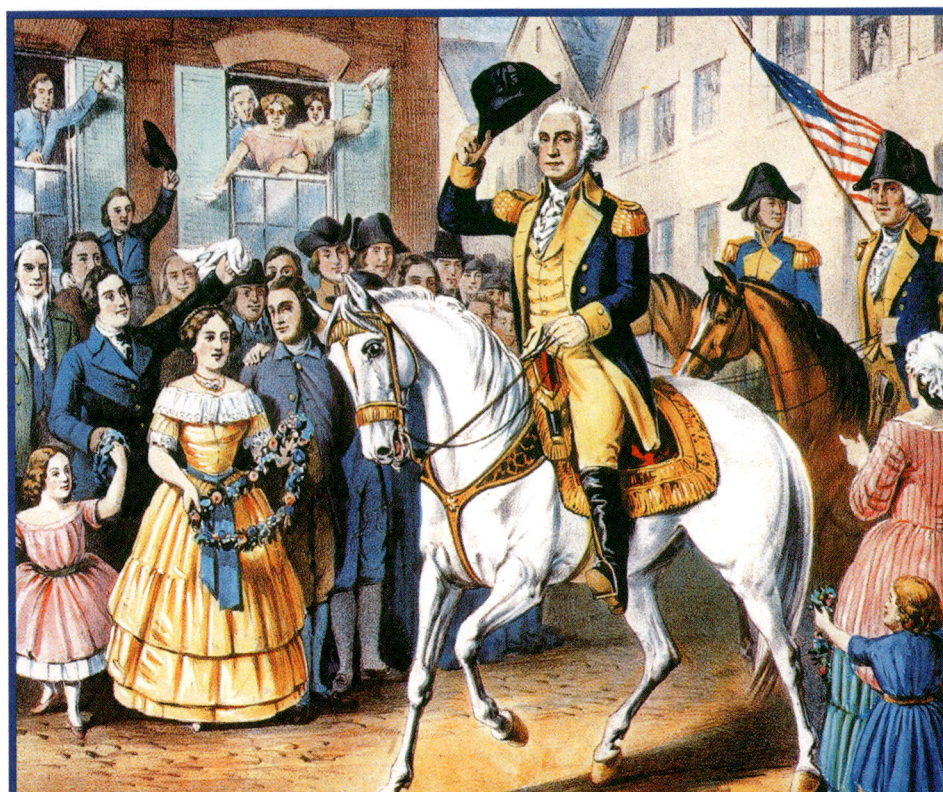

The First Celebration

The first Independence Day was celebrated in 1777 in Philadelphia.

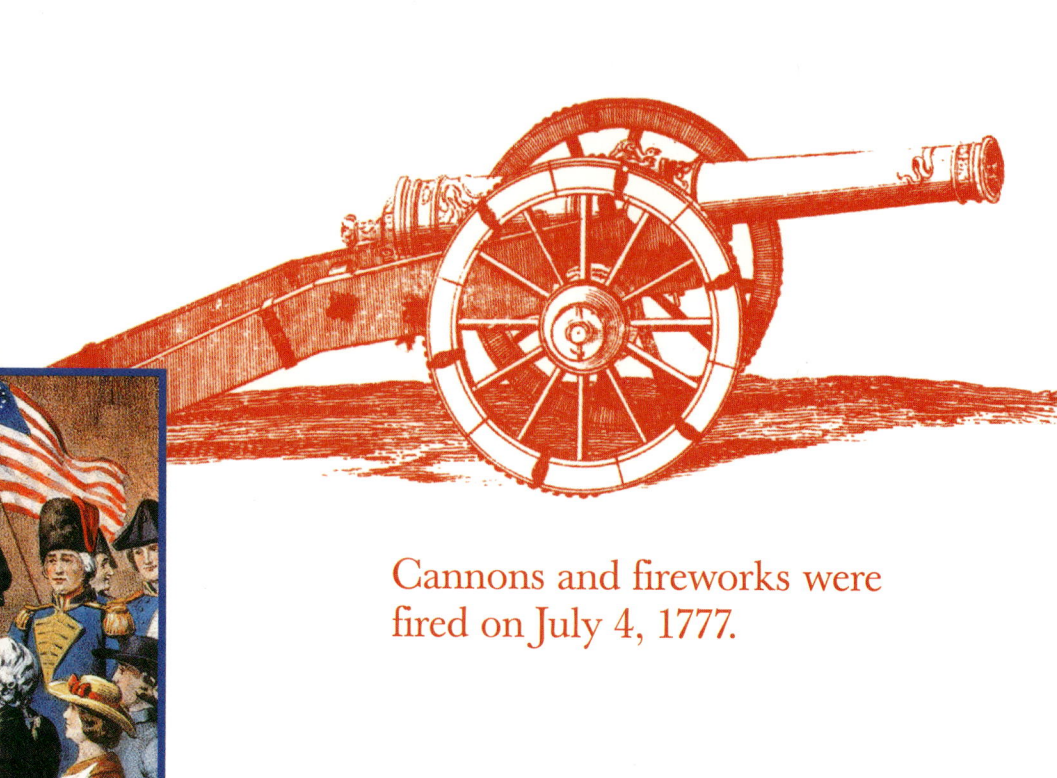

Cannons and fireworks were fired on July 4, 1777.

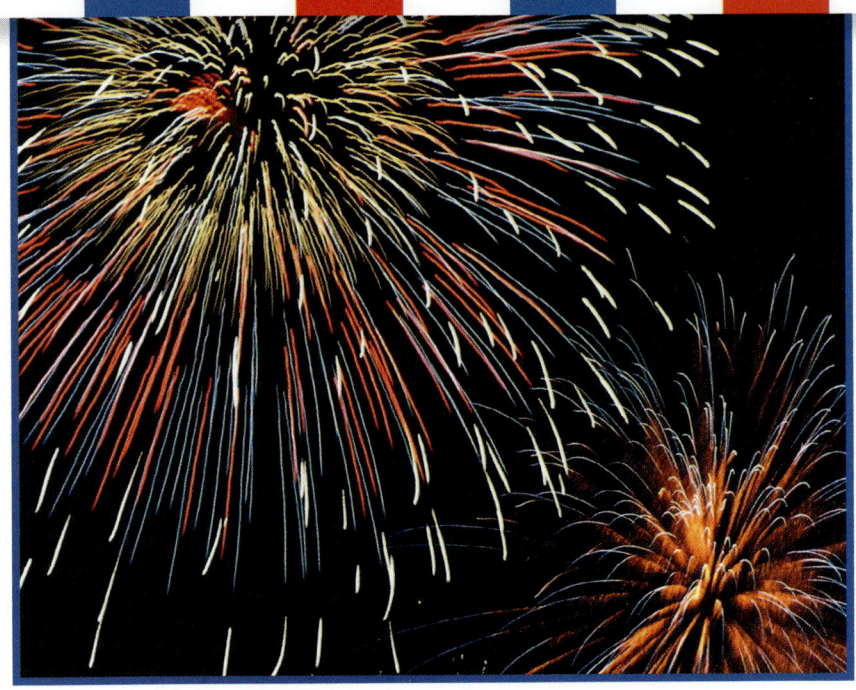

Americans celebrate the Fourth of July with fireworks.

Fireworks

In 1800 New York City celebrated Independence Day with fireworks. American **citizens** loved the fireworks. Later, Boston and some other places began to celebrate with fireworks too!

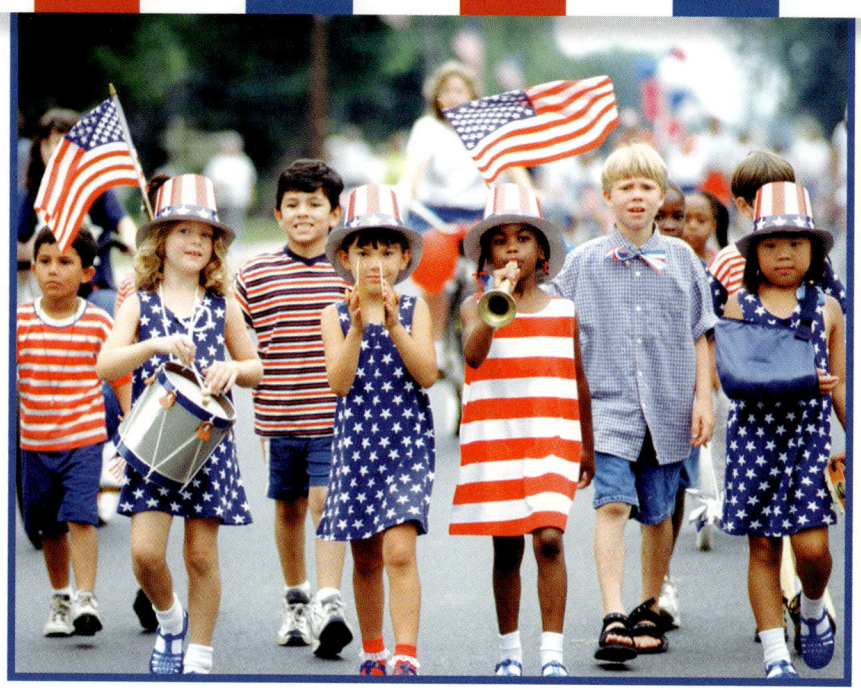

People celebrate the Fourth of July with parades.

Celebrating Today

Today, Americans celebrate Independence Day with parades. Some people wave flags.

At night many people go to see the fireworks. Americans have fun celebrating on July 4.

Glossary

citizen a member of a state and country

colony a place that is ruled by a country that is far away

freedom a person's right to make choices

holiday a special day

President our country's leader

The Fourth of July

by Natalie Goldstein

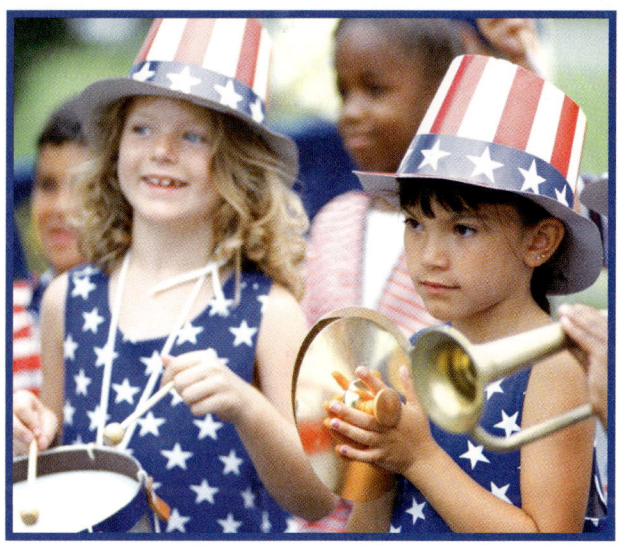

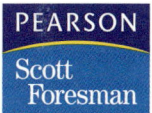

Editorial Offices: Glenview, Illinois • Parsippany, New Jersey • New York, New York
Sales Offices: Needham, Massachusetts • Duluth, Georgia • Glenview, Illinois
Coppell, Texas • Sacramento, California • Mesa, Arizona

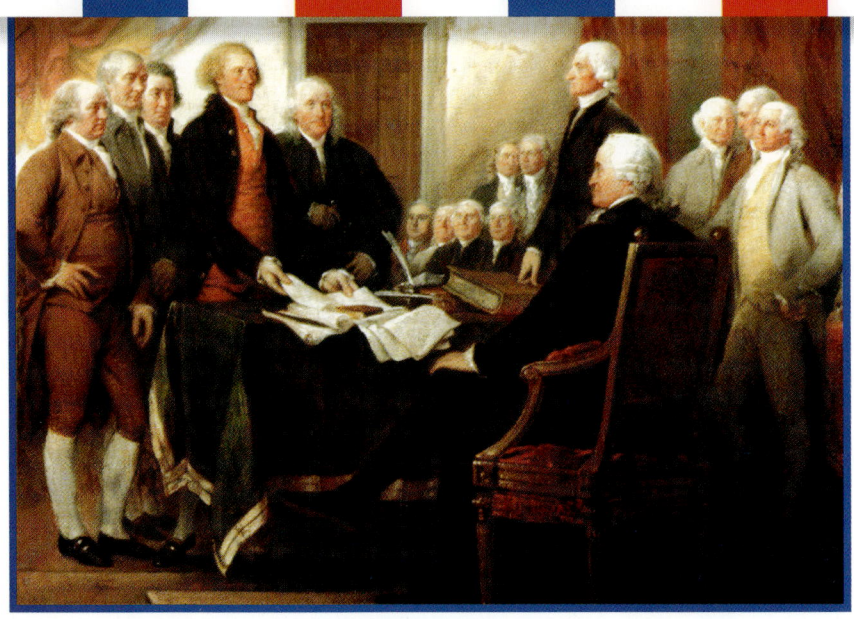

The signing of the Declaration of Independence

The Colonies

Long ago people lived in colonies. The colonies were ruled by England. The colonists wanted **freedom**.

On July 4, 1776, a group of leaders in the colonies agreed on an important paper. It was called the Declaration of Independence.

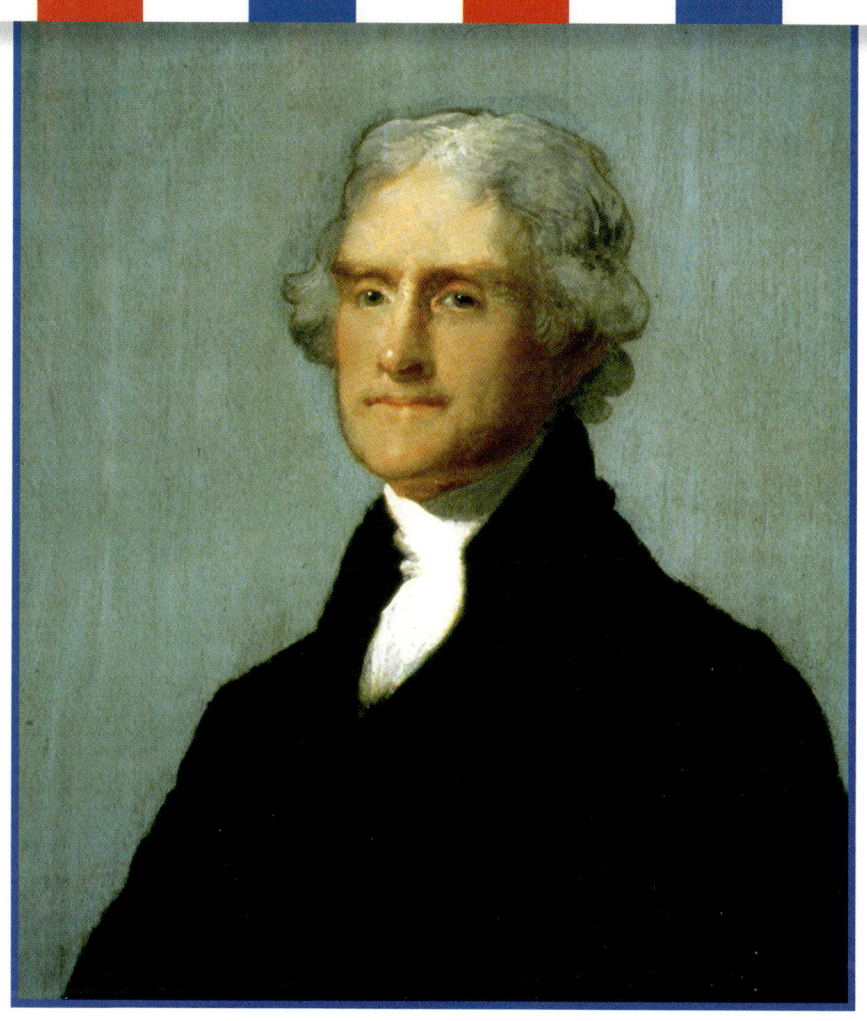

Thomas Jefferson

Most of the Declaration of Independence was written by Thomas Jefferson. July 4 became an American **holiday** to celebrate freedom.

The Fight for Freedom

The colonists had an army to help fight for freedom. George Washington led the army.

The Americans won the war! George Washington became the first **President** of the United States.

George Washington

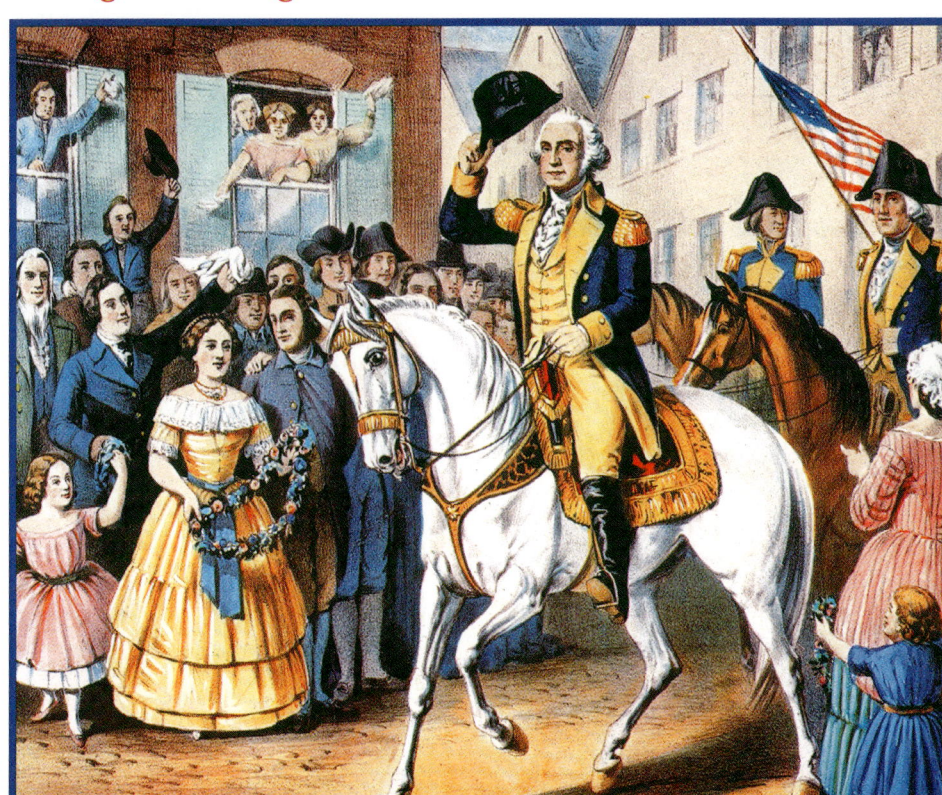

The First Celebration

The first Independence Day was celebrated in 1777 in Philadelphia.

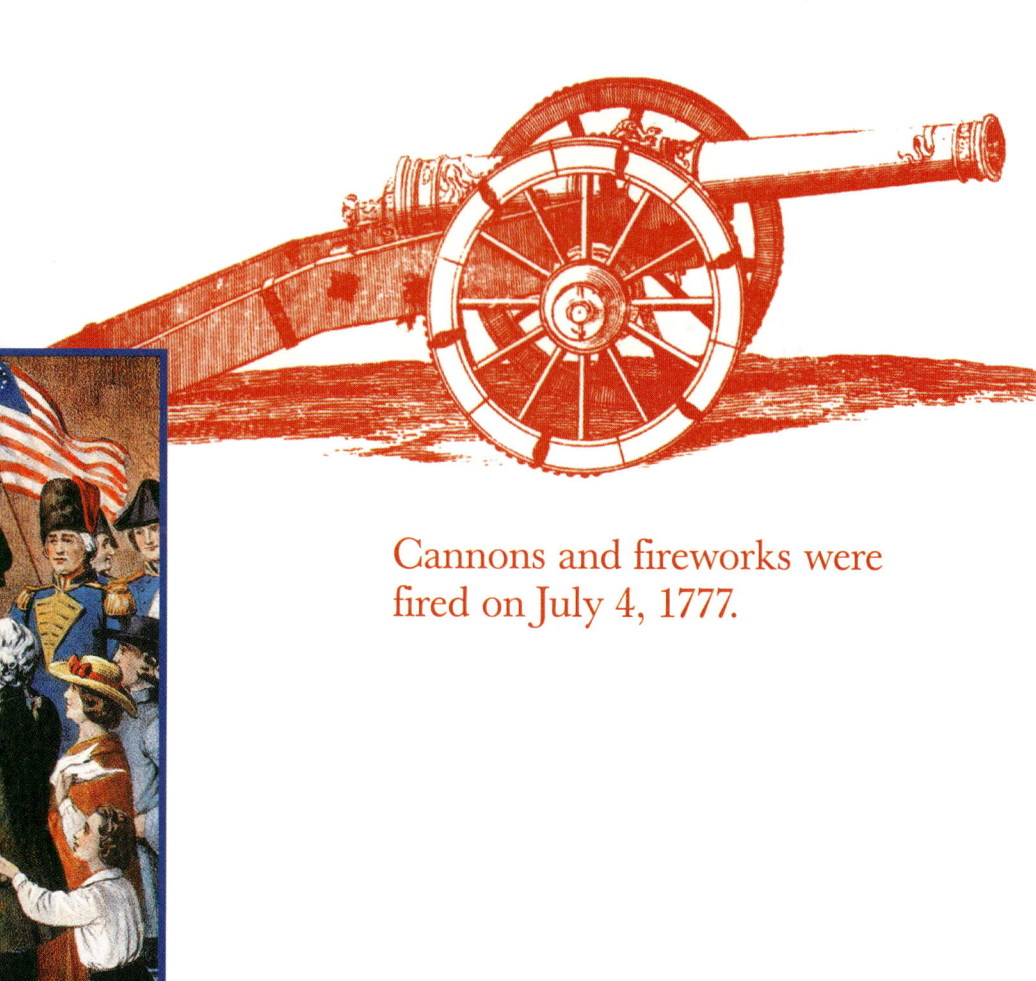

Cannons and fireworks were fired on July 4, 1777.

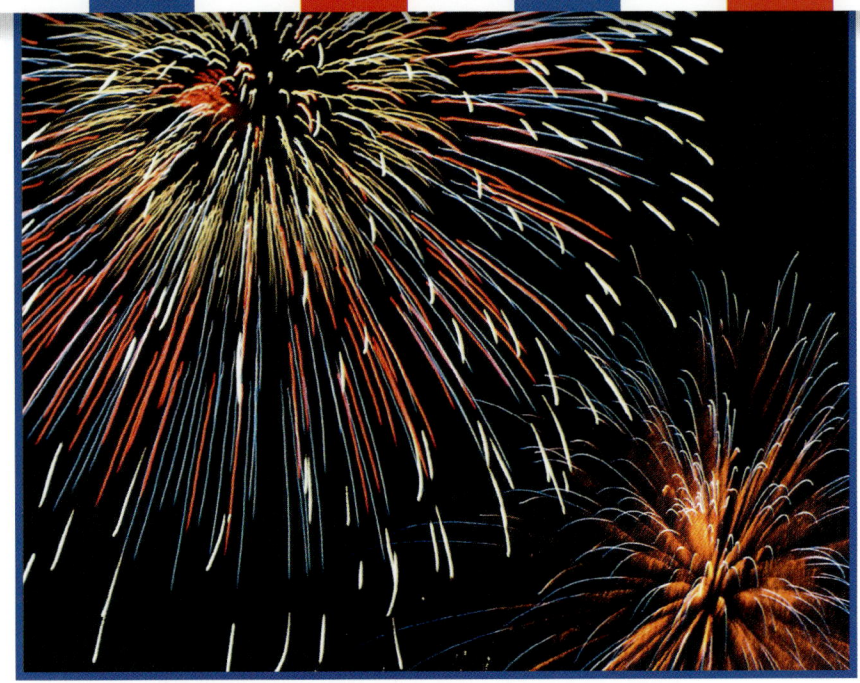

Americans celebrate the Fourth of July with fireworks.

Fireworks

In 1800 New York City celebrated Independence Day with fireworks. American **citizens** loved the fireworks. Later, Boston and some other places began to celebrate with fireworks too!

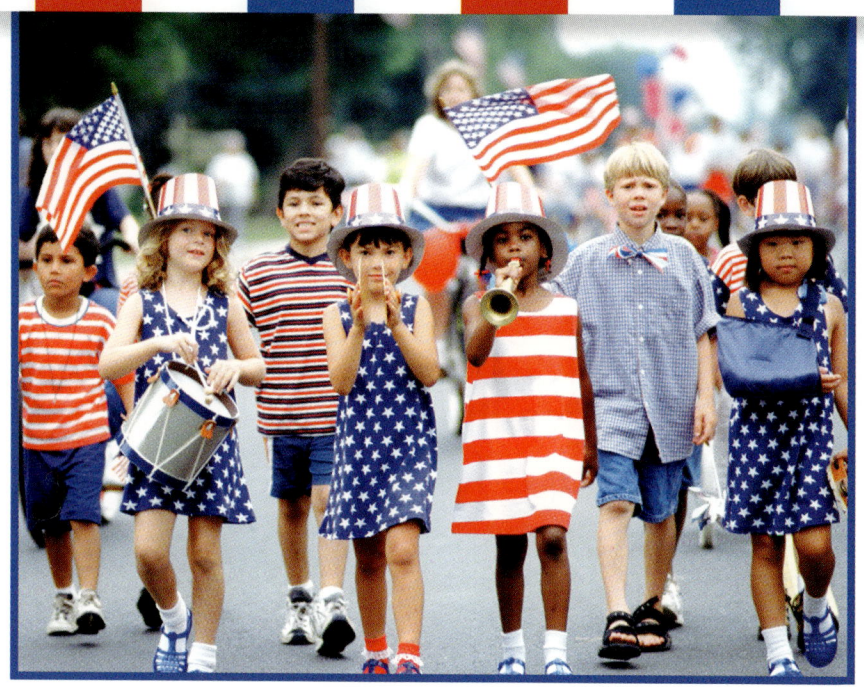

People celebrate the Fourth of July with parades.

Celebrating Today

Today, Americans celebrate Independence Day with parades. Some people wave flags.

At night many people go to see the fireworks. Americans have fun celebrating on July 4.

Glossary

citizen a member of a state and country

colony a place that is ruled by a country that is far away

freedom a person's right to make choices

holiday a special day

President our country's leader

The Fourth of July

by Natalie Goldstein

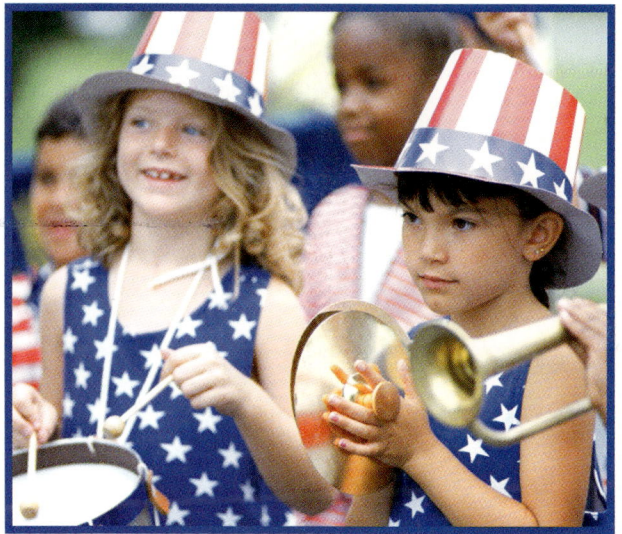

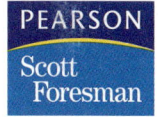

Editorial Offices: Glenview, Illinois • Parsippany, New Jersey • New York, New York
Sales Offices: Needham, Massachusetts • Duluth, Georgia • Glenview, Illinois
Coppell, Texas • Sacramento, California • Mesa, Arizona

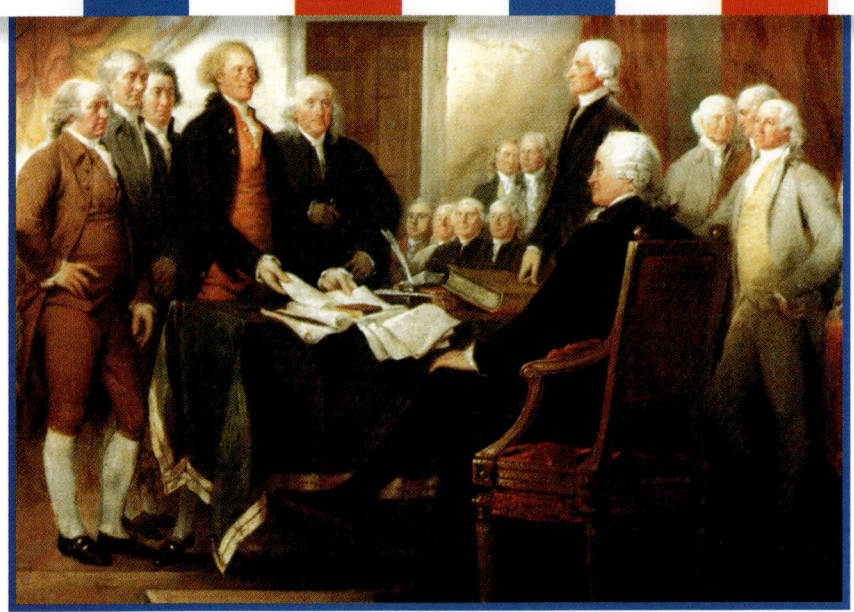

The signing of the Declaration of Independence

The Colonies

Long ago people lived in colonies. The colonies were ruled by England. The colonists wanted **freedom**.

On July 4, 1776, a group of leaders in the colonies agreed on an important paper. It was called the Declaration of Independence.

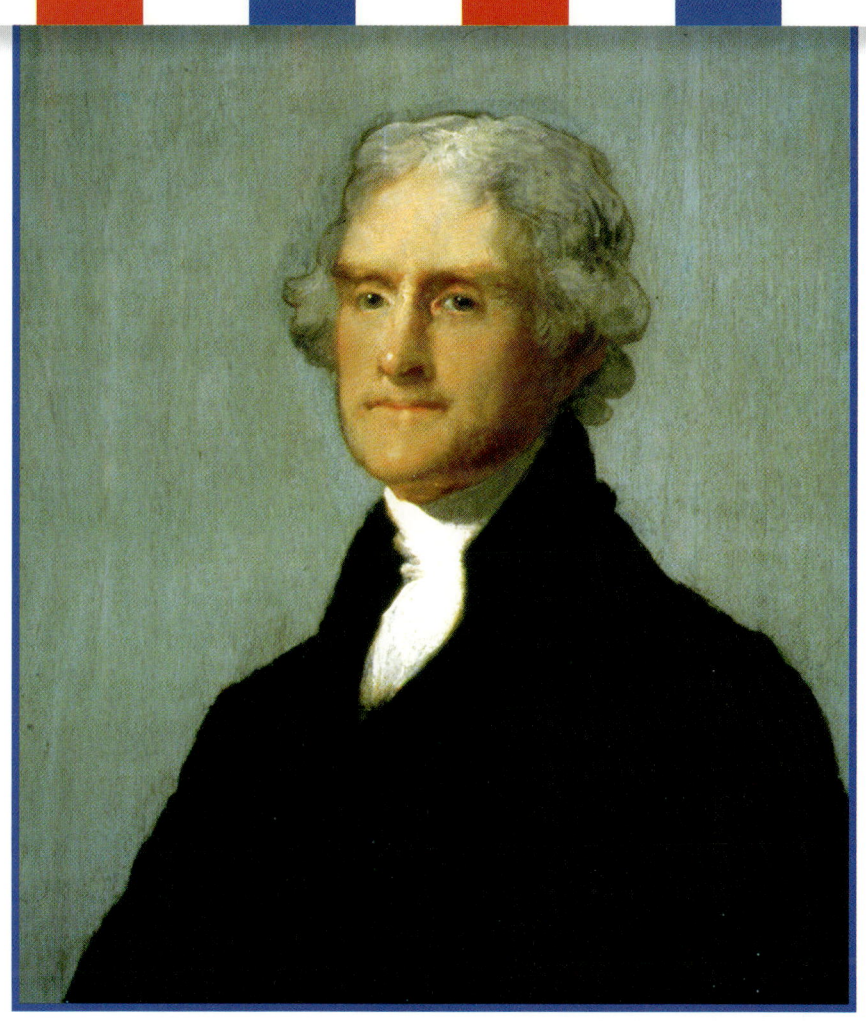

Thomas Jefferson

Most of the Declaration of Independence was written by Thomas Jefferson. July 4 became an American **holiday** to celebrate freedom.

The Fight for Freedom

The colonists had an army to help fight for freedom. George Washington led the army.

The Americans won the war! George Washington became the first **President** of the United States.

George Washington

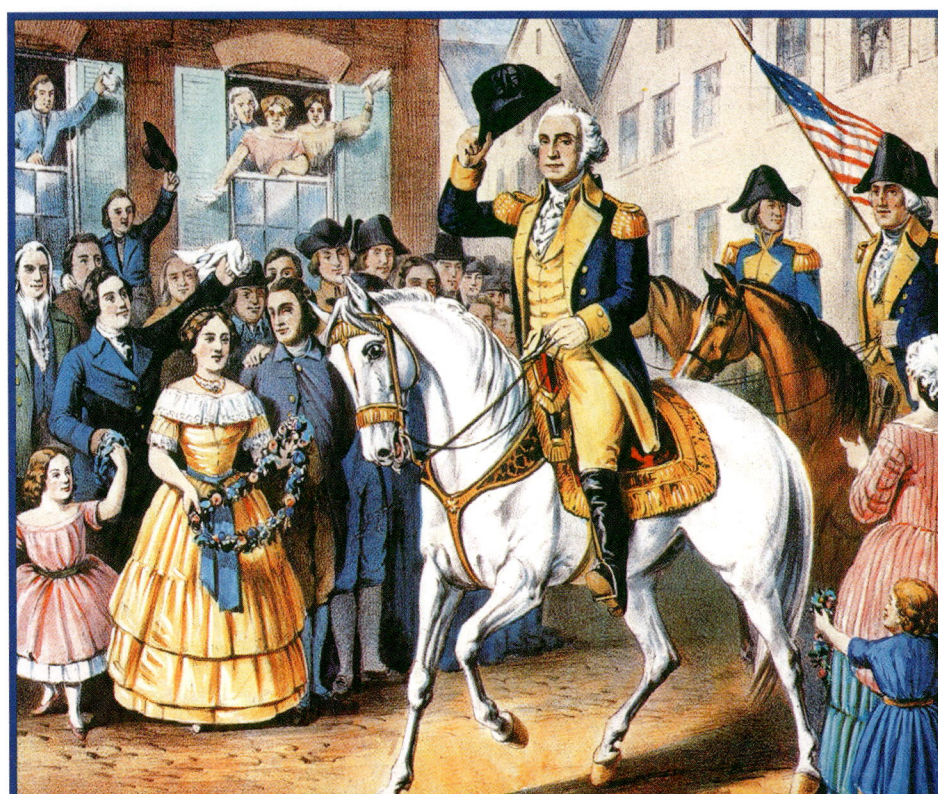

The First Celebration

The first Independence Day was celebrated in 1777 in Philadelphia.

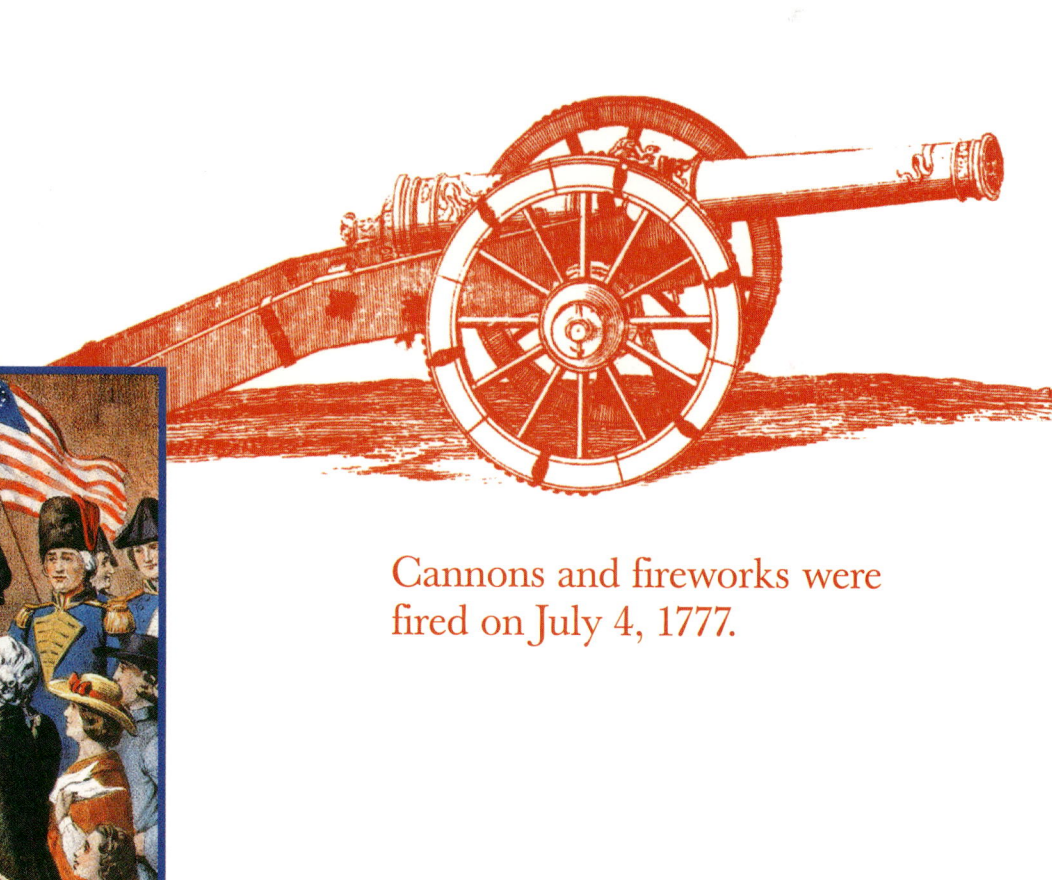

Cannons and fireworks were fired on July 4, 1777.

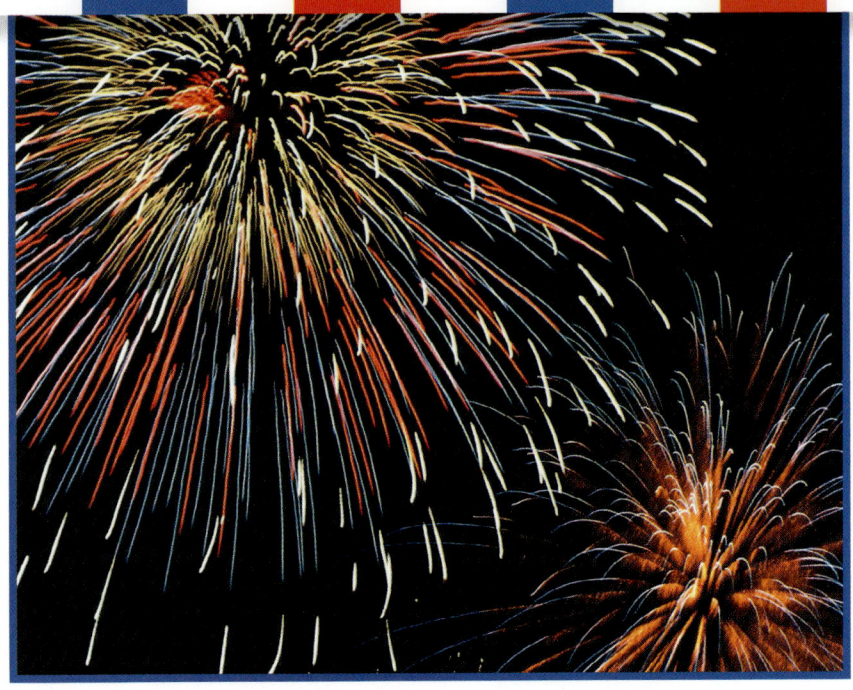

Americans celebrate the Fourth of July with fireworks.

Fireworks

In 1800 New York City celebrated Independence Day with fireworks. American **citizens** loved the fireworks. Later, Boston and some other places began to celebrate with fireworks too!

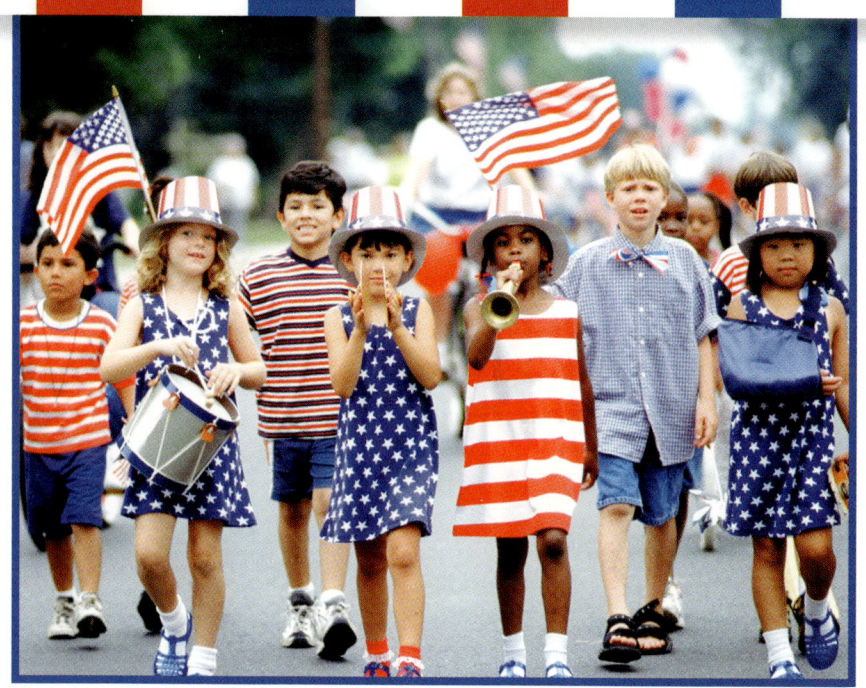

People celebrate the Fourth of July with parades.

Celebrating Today

Today, Americans celebrate Independence Day with parades. Some people wave flags.

At night many people go to see the fireworks. Americans have fun celebrating on July 4.

Glossary

citizen a member of a state and country

colony a place that is ruled by a country that is far away

freedom a person's right to make choices

holiday a special day

President our country's leader

The Fourth of July

by Natalie Goldstein

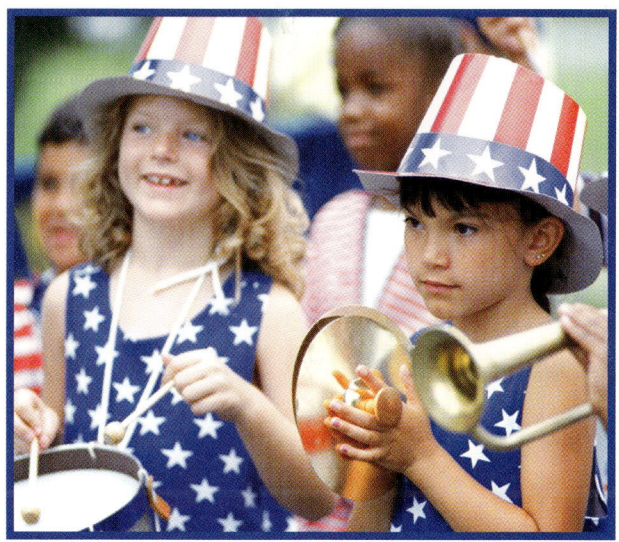

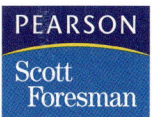

Editorial Offices: Glenview, Illinois • Parsippany, New Jersey • New York, New York
Sales Offices: Needham, Massachusetts • Duluth, Georgia • Glenview, Illinois
Coppell, Texas • Sacramento, California • Mesa, Arizona

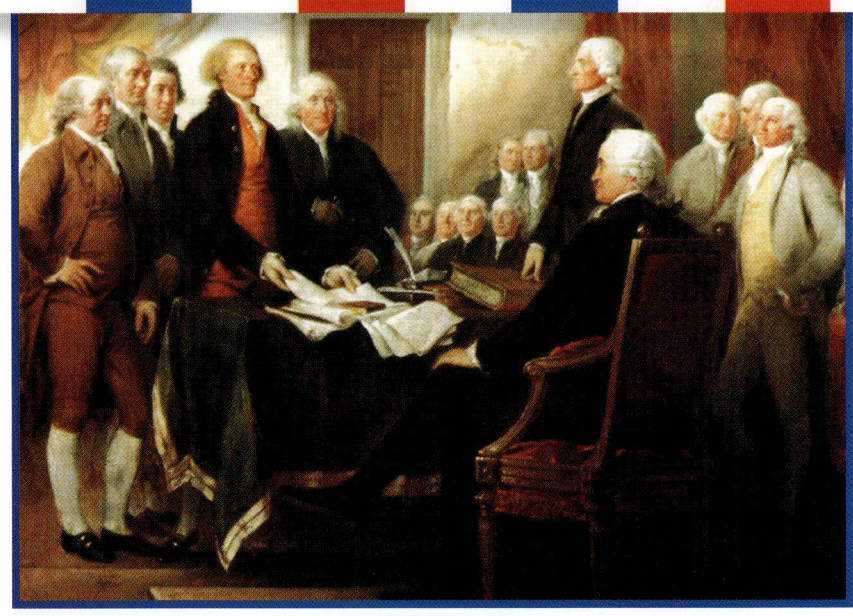

The signing of the Declaration of Independence

The Colonies

Long ago people lived in colonies. The colonies were ruled by England. The colonists wanted **freedom**.

On July 4, 1776, a group of leaders in the colonies agreed on an important paper. It was called the Declaration of Independence.

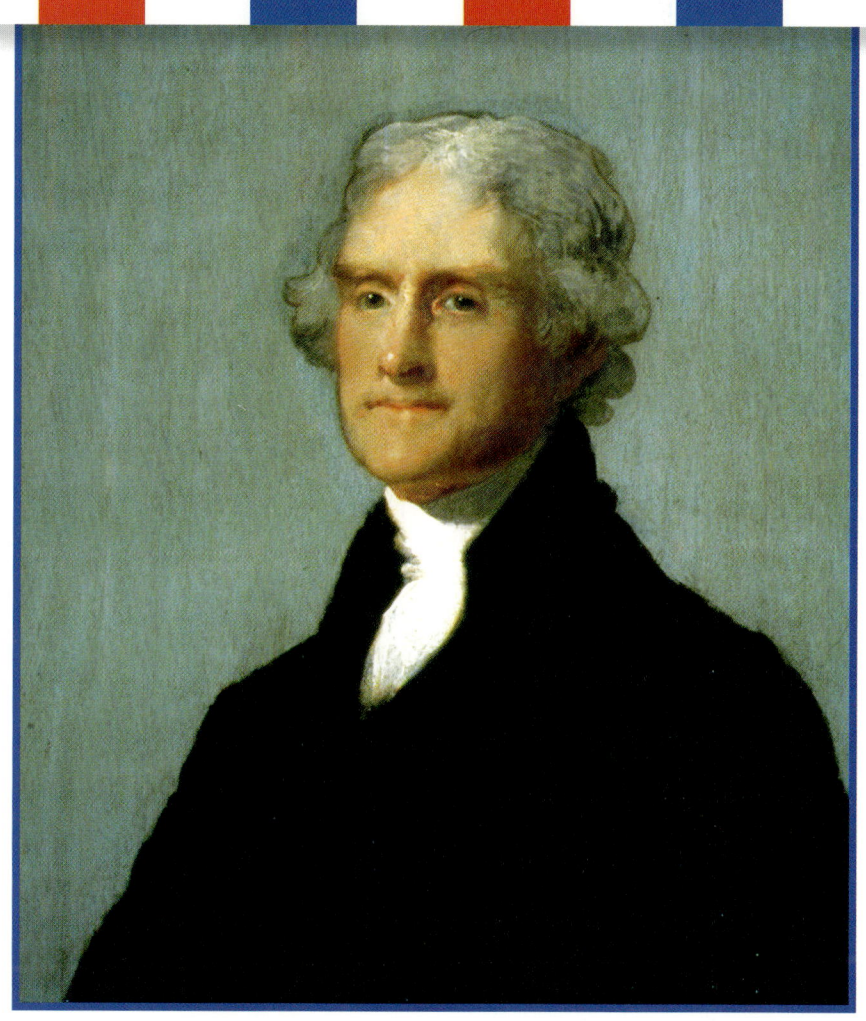

Thomas Jefferson

Most of the Declaration of Independence was written by Thomas Jefferson. July 4 became an American **holiday** to celebrate freedom.

The Fight for Freedom

The colonists had an army to help fight for freedom. George Washington led the army.

The Americans won the war! George Washington became the first **President** of the United States.

George Washington

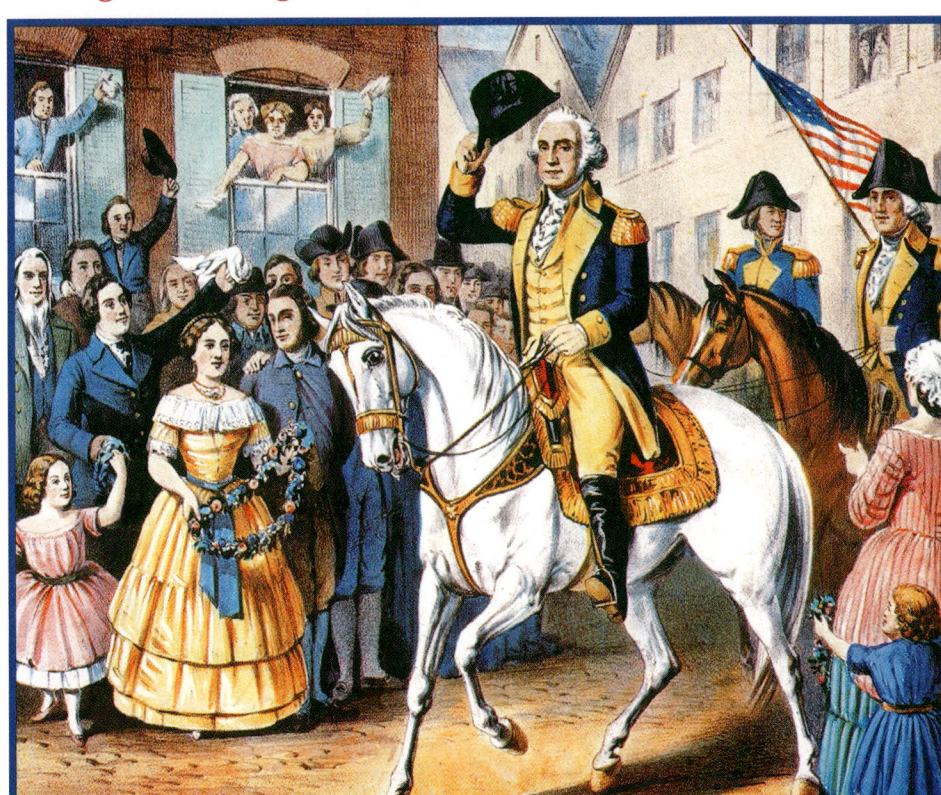

The First Celebration

The first Independence Day was celebrated in 1777 in Philadelphia.

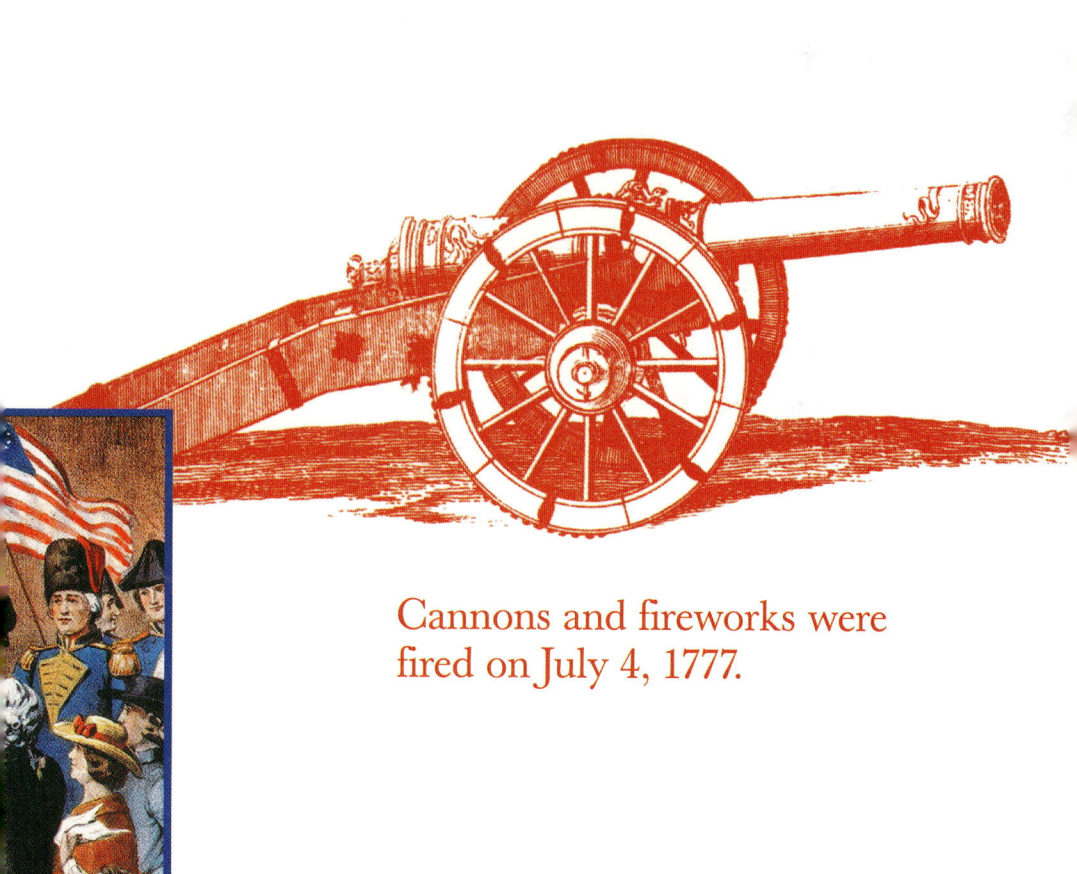

Cannons and fireworks were fired on July 4, 1777.

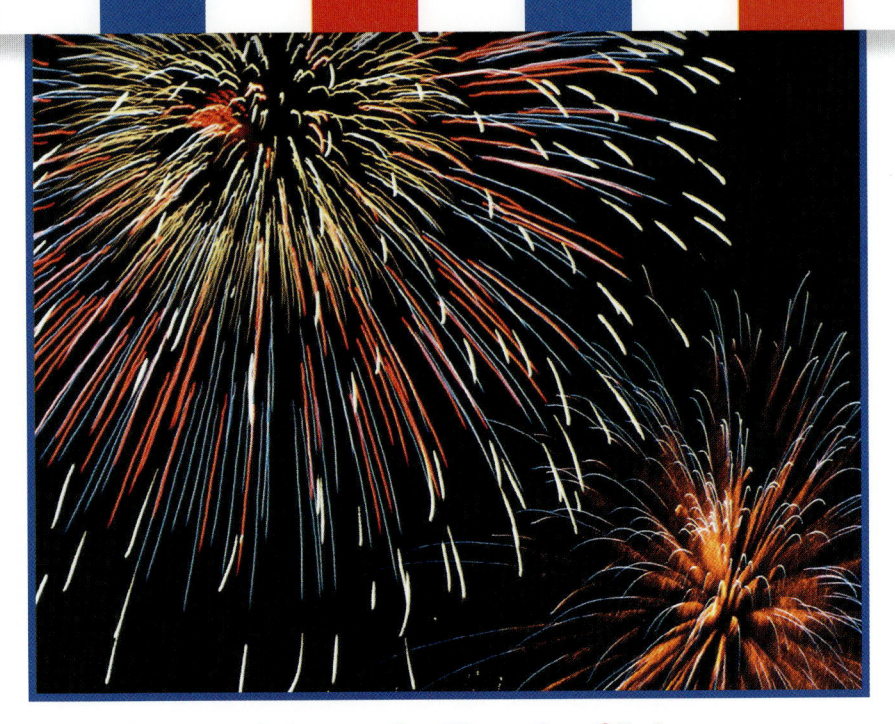

Americans celebrate the Fourth of July with fireworks.

Fireworks

In 1800 New York City celebrated Independence Day with fireworks. American **citizens** loved the fireworks. Later, Boston and some other places began to celebrate with fireworks too!

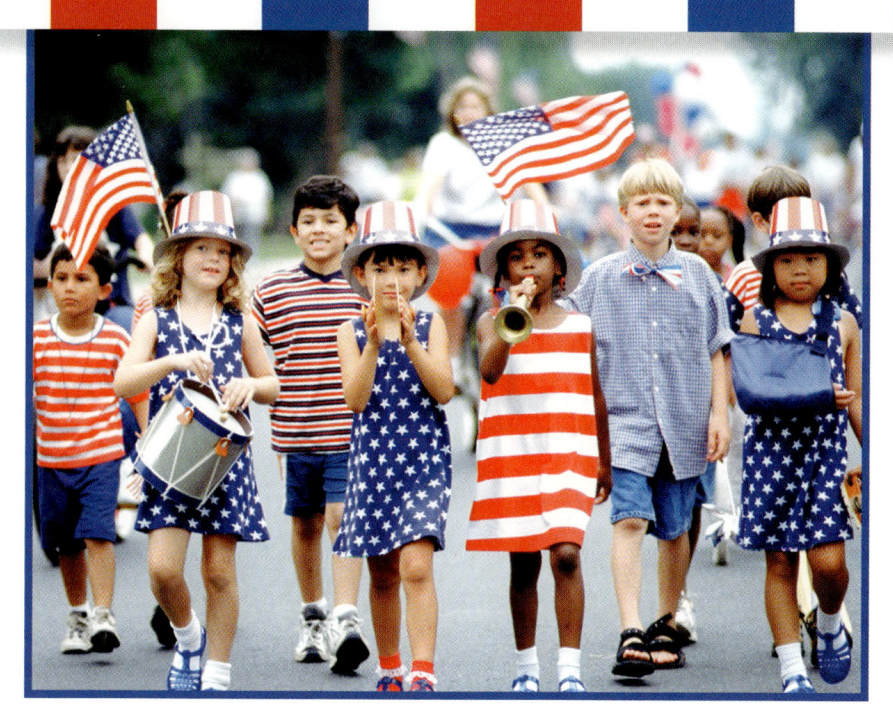

People celebrate the Fourth of July with parades.

Celebrating Today

Today, Americans celebrate Independence Day with parades. Some people wave flags.

At night many people go to see the fireworks. Americans have fun celebrating on July 4.

Glossary

citizen a member of a state and country

colony a place that is ruled by a country that is far away

freedom a person's right to make choices

holiday a special day

President our country's leader

The Fourth of July

by Natalie Goldstein

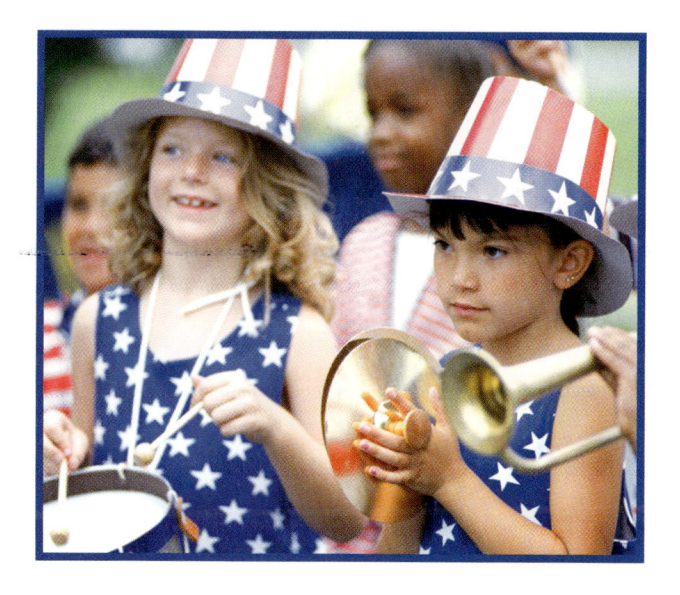

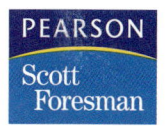

PEARSON
Scott Foresman

Editorial Offices: Glenview, Illinois • Parsippany, New Jersey • New York, New York
Sales Offices: Needham, Massachusetts • Duluth, Georgia • Glenview, Illinois
Coppell, Texas • Sacramento, California • Mesa, Arizona

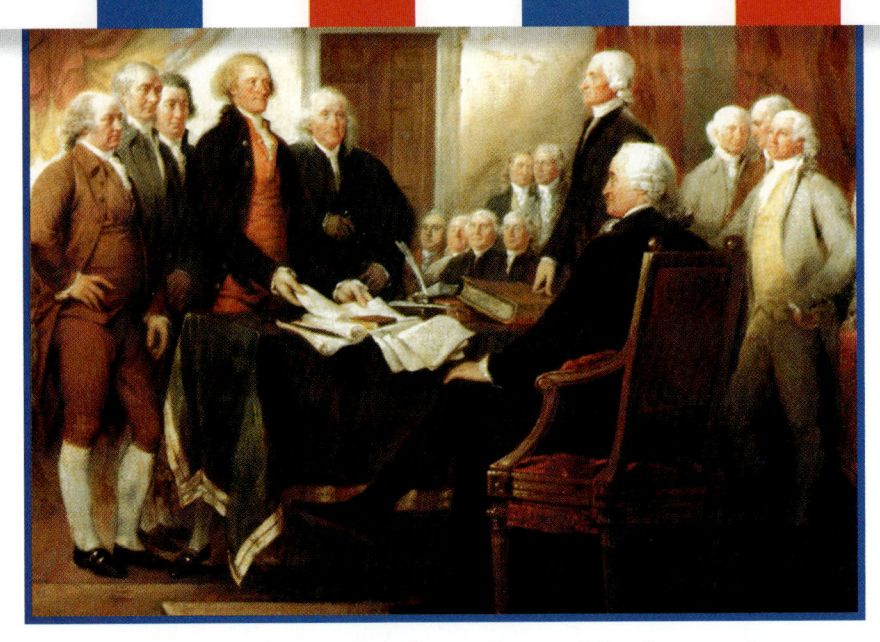

The signing of the Declaration of Independence

The Colonies

Long ago people lived in colonies. The colonies were ruled by England. The colonists wanted **freedom**.

On July 4, 1776, a group of leaders in the colonies agreed on an important paper. It was called the Declaration of Independence.

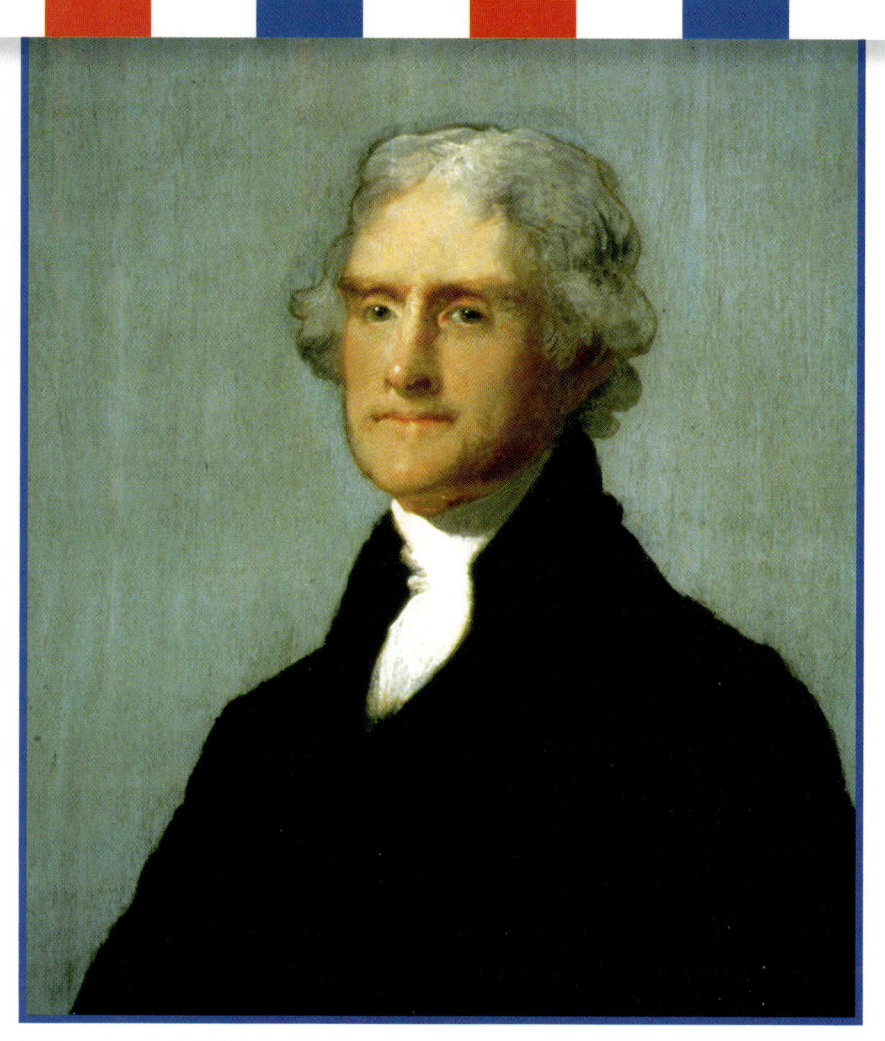

Thomas Jefferson

Most of the Declaration of Independence was written by Thomas Jefferson. July 4 became an American **holiday** to celebrate freedom.

The Fight for Freedom

The colonists had an army to help fight for freedom. George Washington led the army.

The Americans won the war! George Washington became the first **President** of the United States.

George Washington

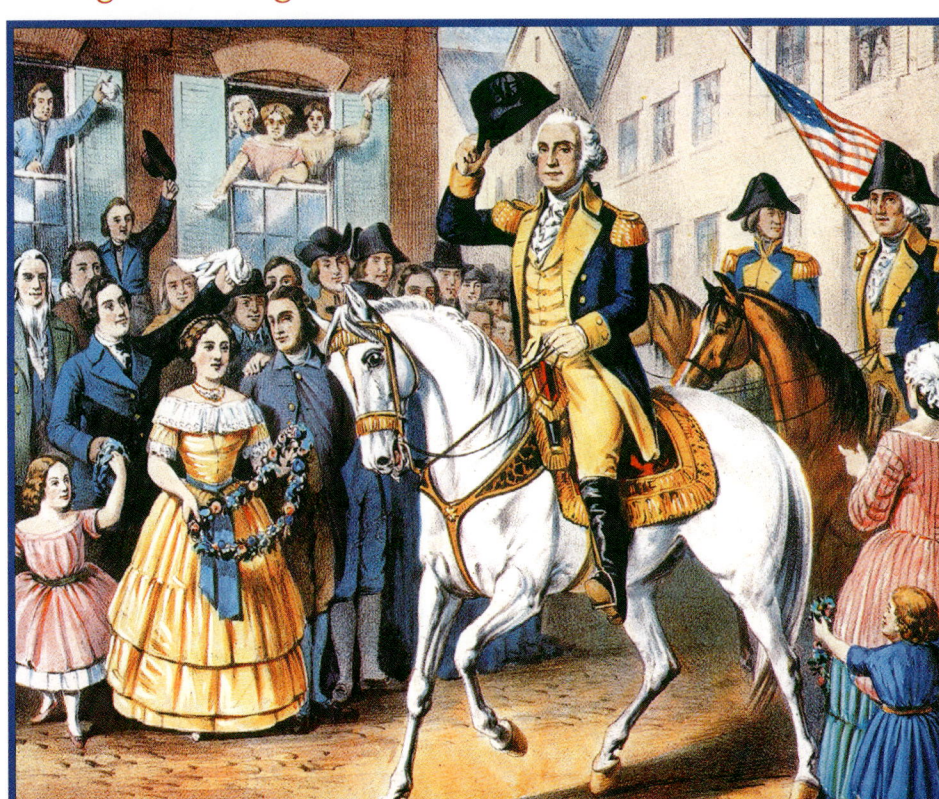

The First Celebration

The first Independence Day was celebrated in 1777 in Philadelphia.

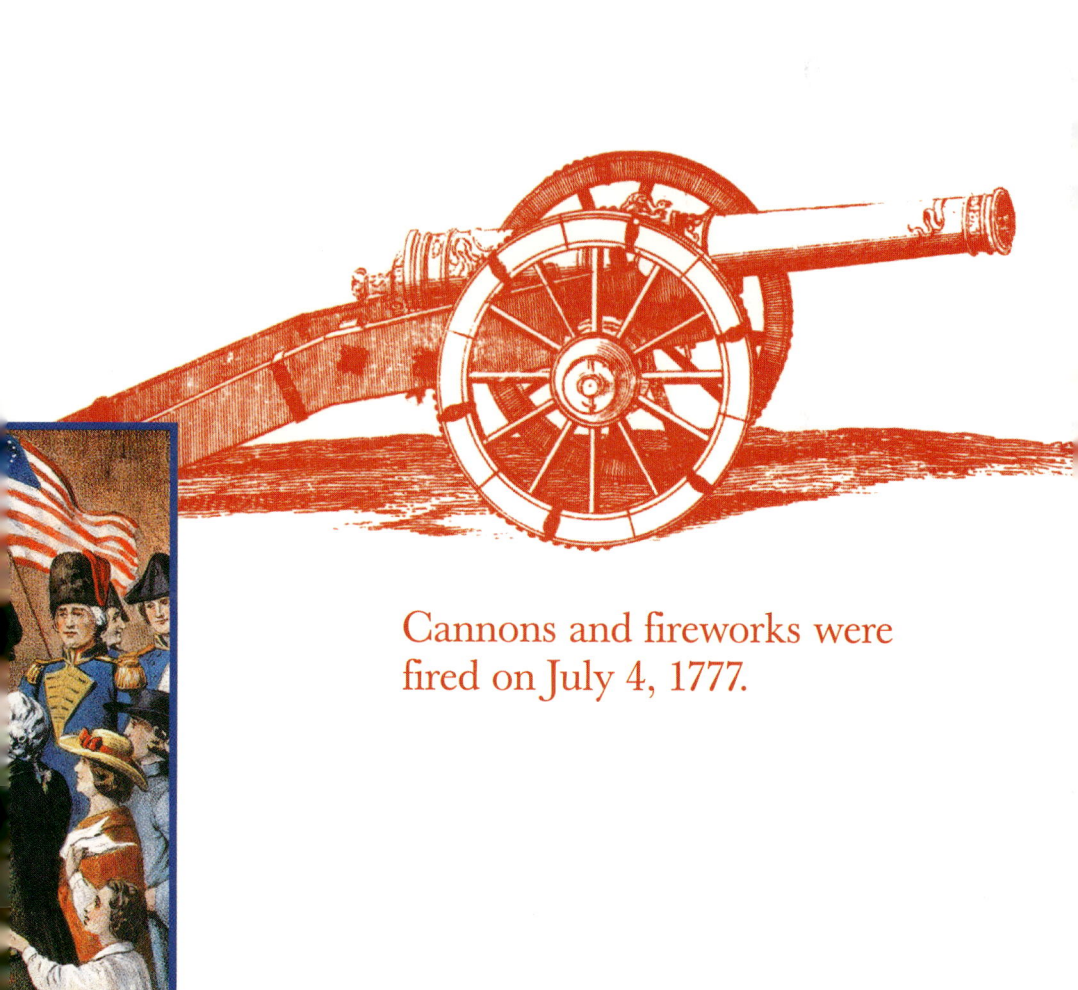

Cannons and fireworks were fired on July 4, 1777.

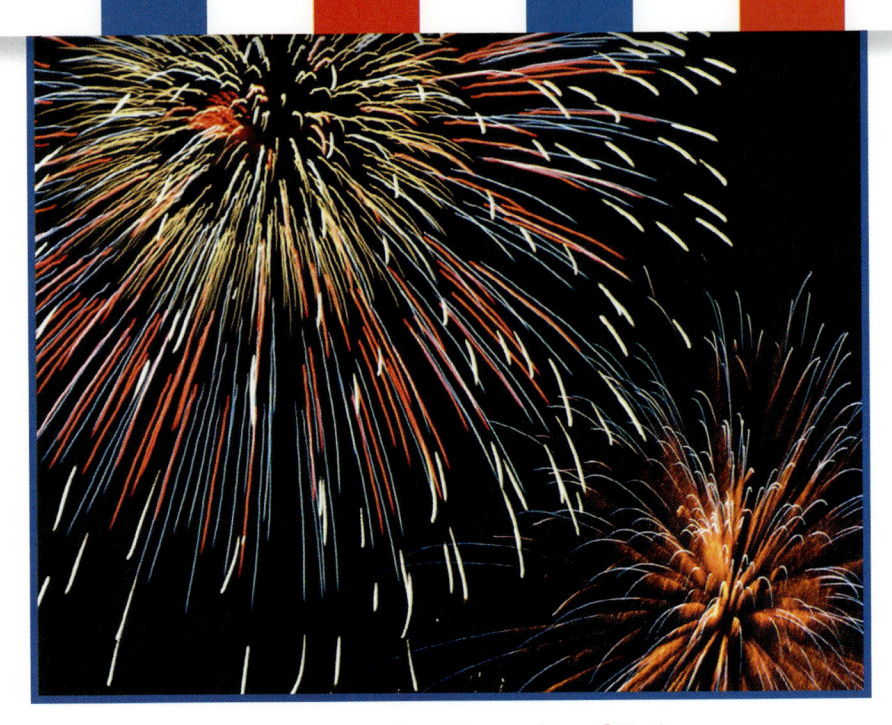

Americans celebrate the Fourth of July with fireworks.

Fireworks

In 1800 New York City celebrated Independence Day with fireworks. American **citizens** loved the fireworks. Later, Boston and some other places began to celebrate with fireworks too!

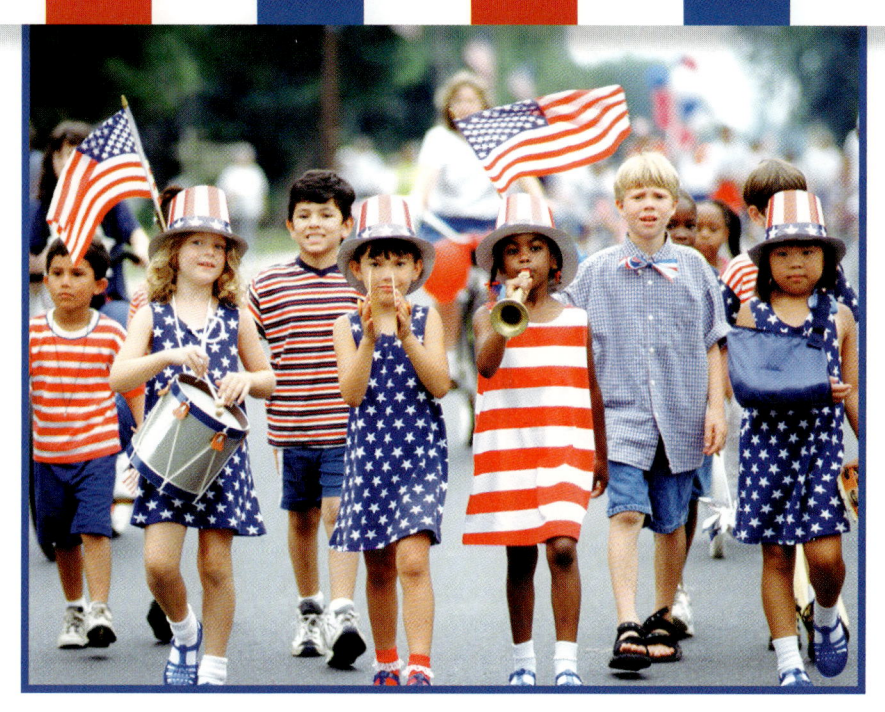

People celebrate the Fourth of July with parades.

Celebrating Today

Today, Americans celebrate Independence Day with parades. Some people wave flags.

At night many people go to see the fireworks. Americans have fun celebrating on July 4.

Glossary

citizen a member of a state and country

colony a place that is ruled by a country that is far away

freedom a person's right to make choices

holiday a special day

President our country's leader

The Fourth of July

by Natalie Goldstein

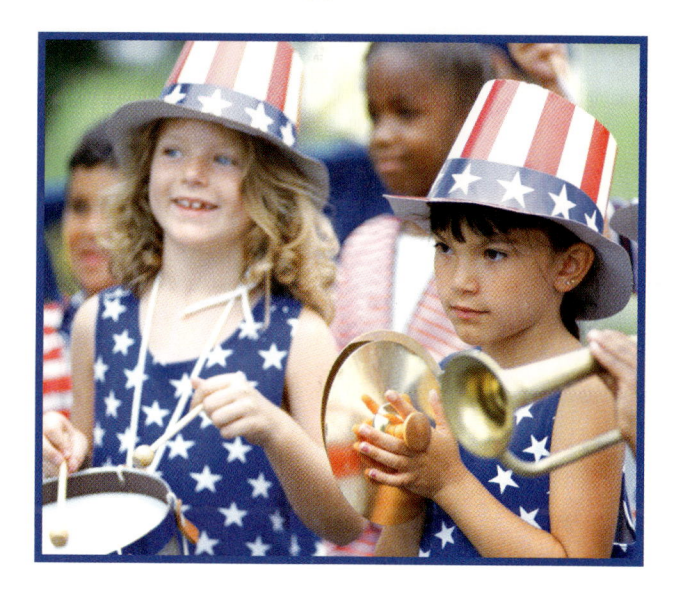

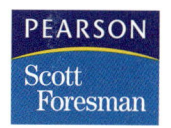

PEARSON
Scott Foresman

Editorial Offices: Glenview, Illinois • Parsippany, New Jersey • New York, New York
Sales Offices: Needham, Massachusetts • Duluth, Georgia • Glenview, Illinois
Coppell, Texas • Sacramento, California • Mesa, Arizona

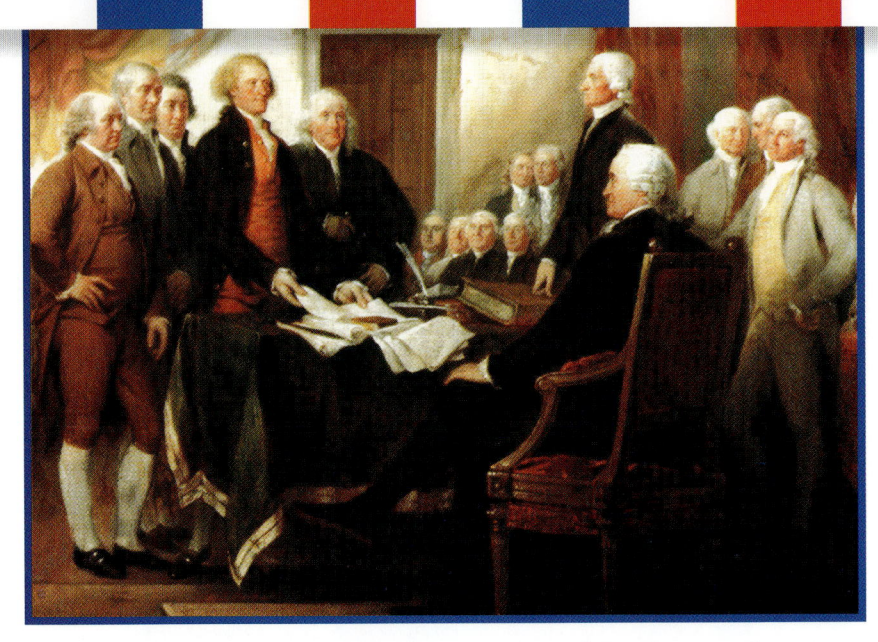

The signing of the Declaration of Independence

The Colonies

Long ago people lived in colonies. The colonies were ruled by England. The colonists wanted **freedom**.

On July 4, 1776, a group of leaders in the colonies agreed on an important paper. It was called the Declaration of Independence.

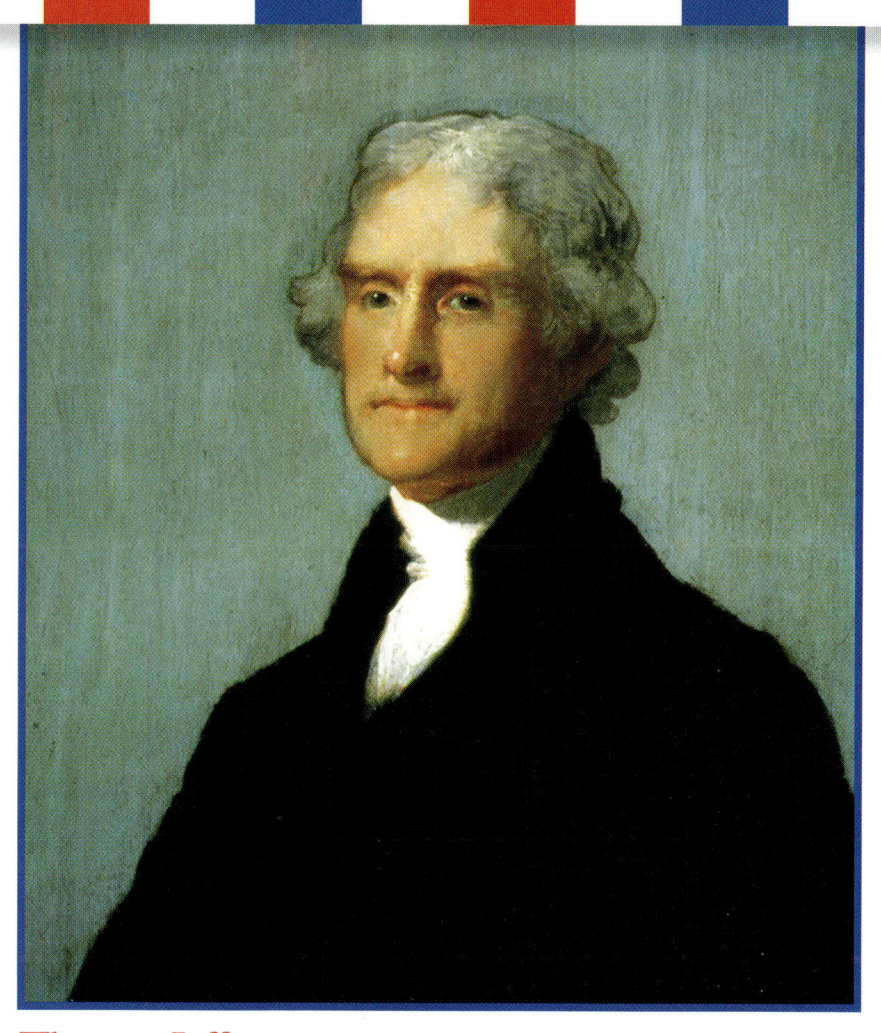

Thomas Jefferson

Most of the Declaration of Independence was written by Thomas Jefferson. July 4 became an American **holiday** to celebrate freedom.

The Fight for Freedom

The colonists had an army to help fight for freedom. George Washington led the army.

The Americans won the war! George Washington became the first **President** of the United States.

George Washington

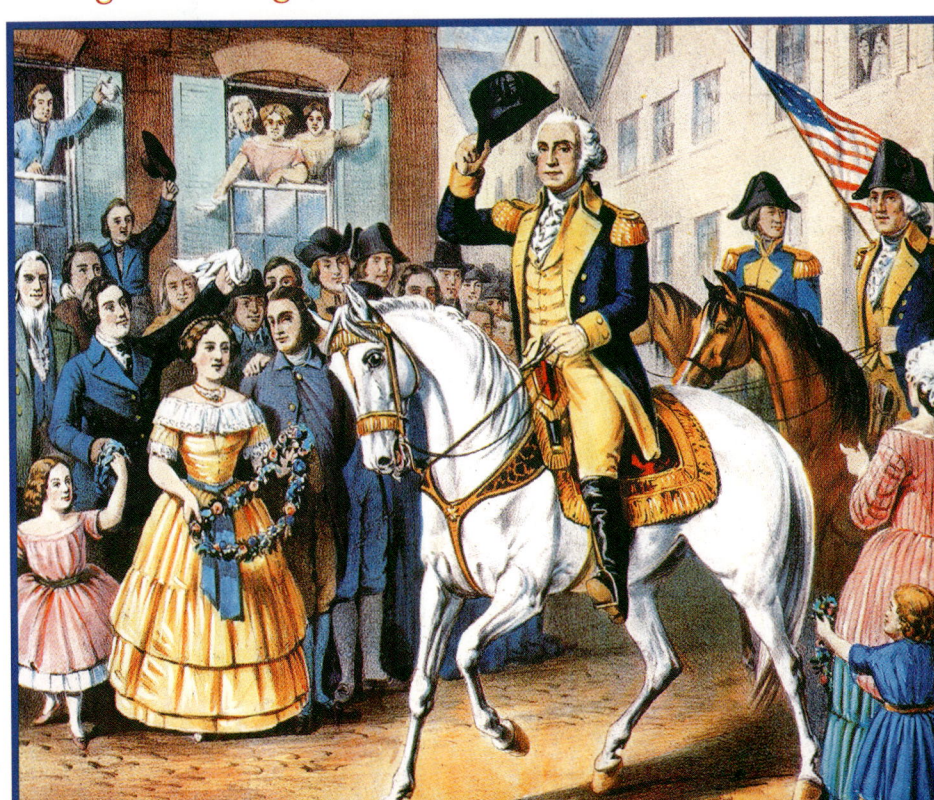

The First Celebration

The first Independence Day was celebrated in 1777 in Philadelphia.

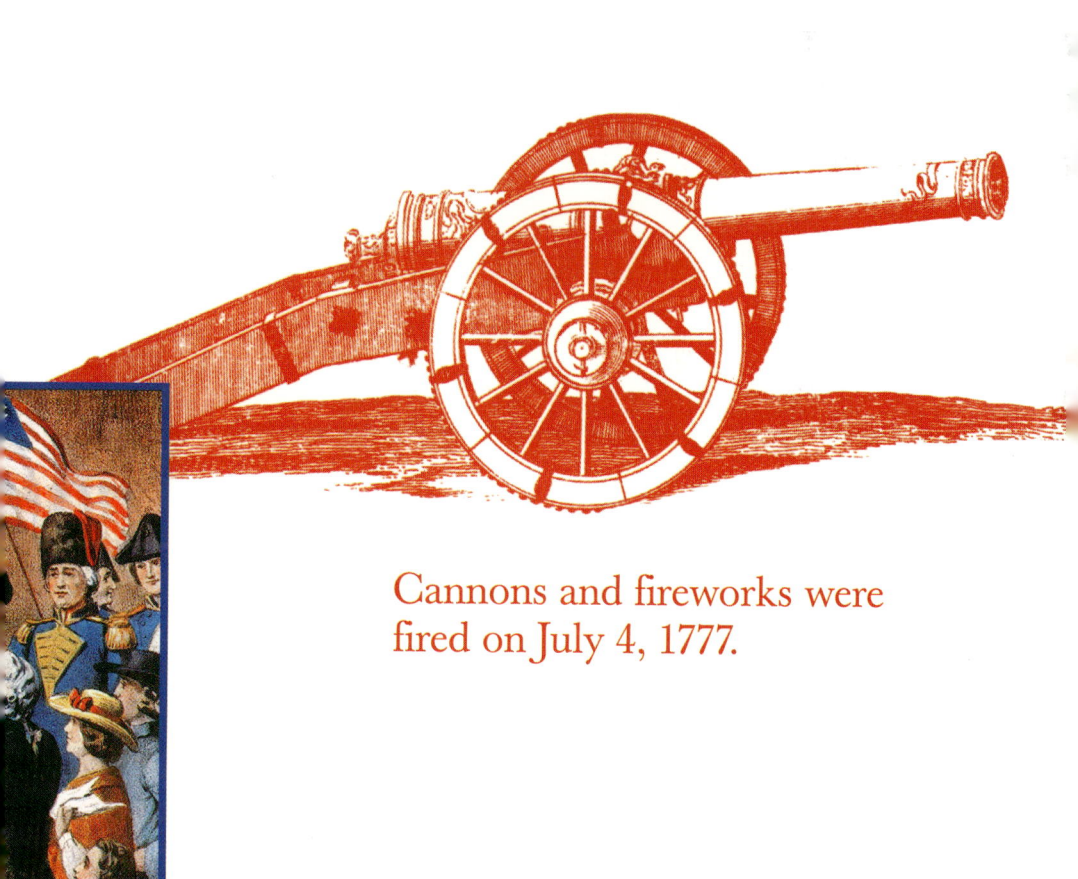

Cannons and fireworks were fired on July 4, 1777.

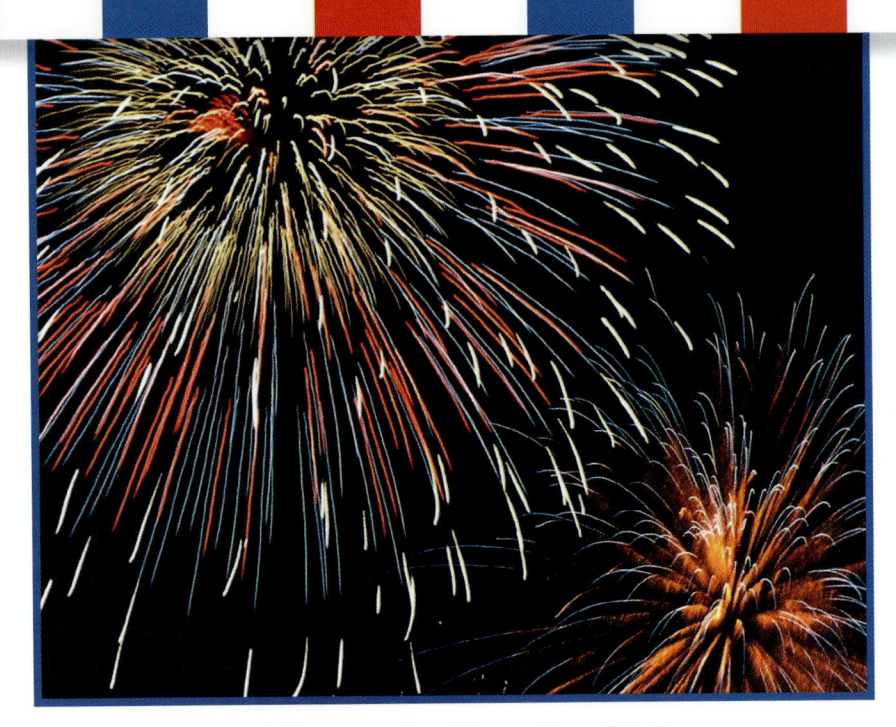

Americans celebrate the Fourth of July with fireworks.

Fireworks

In 1800 New York City celebrated Independence Day with fireworks. American **citizens** loved the fireworks. Later, Boston and some other places began to celebrate with fireworks too!

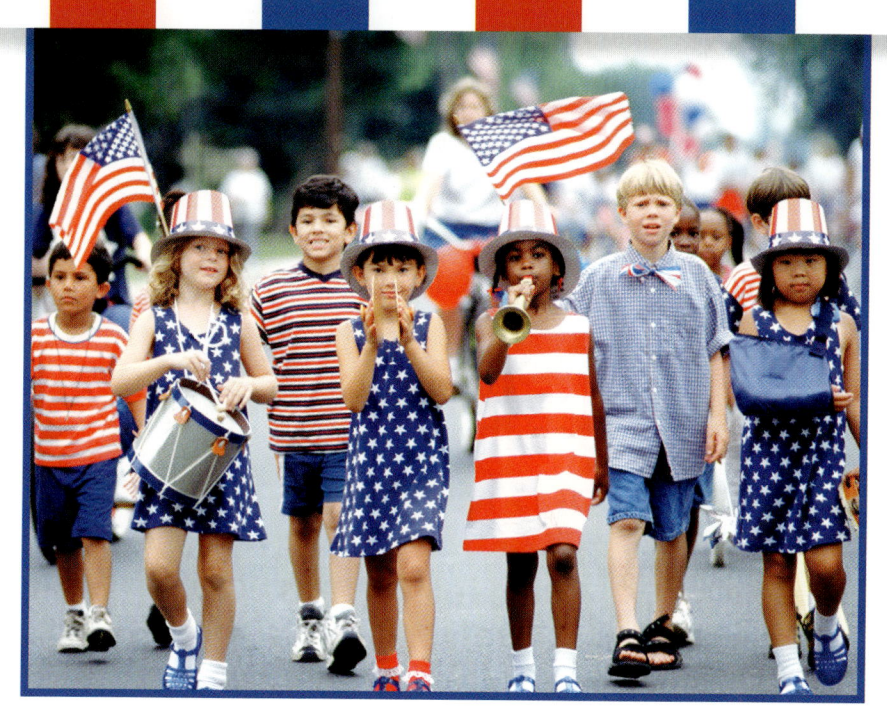

People celebrate the Fourth of July with parades.

Celebrating Today

Today, Americans celebrate Independence Day with parades. Some people wave flags.

At night many people go to see the fireworks. Americans have fun celebrating on July 4.

Glossary

citizen a member of a state and country

colony a place that is ruled by a country that is far away

freedom a person's right to make choices

holiday a special day

President our country's leader